PERSPECTIVE

PERSPECTIVE

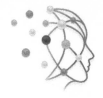

REWIRE YOUR **BRAIN** FOR
SUCCESS AND ABUNDANCE

DR. CHRIS BOMAN

PERSPECTIVE
Rewire Your Brain for Success and Abundance

ISBN   978-1-5445-2773-4   *Hardcover*

        978-1-5445-2771-0   *Paperback*

        978-1-5445-2772-7   *Ebook*

CONTENTS

DISCLAIMER

A WORD OF CAUTION: THIS BOOK SHOULD IN NO WAY BE USED AS a replacement for medical care. I am not a medical doctor, pediatrician, gastroenterologist, neuroscientist, or psychiatrist. If you believe you are experiencing a life-threatening medical condition that requires attention or treatment, you should seek immediate assistance. No book can diagnose or treat a specific ailment or condition.

FOREWORD

—*Peter Voogd*

THE SHIFT IN PERSPECTIVE ADVOCATED BY CHRIS BOMAN IS something I've been advocating for a long time. Understanding the power of one perspective shift (and the different ways we can all view any given situation) can yield a totally different life, a totally different success story, and a totally different income stream. One way that Dr. Chris's book really stands out is that he mixes research, clinical studies, and his years of being in the trenches not just as a chiropractor but also as an entrepreneur, building a successful practice from scratch. His combined experience makes for an amazing book that I really believe can change people's lives. It's a change we all need more than ever, particularly as health concerns increase and we move towards the new economy.

This is a subject I am personally committed to. I've written three best-selling books, and I've spent a quarter-million dollars on my own personal growth and business journey. When it comes to investing in myself, I am extremely serious about educating my mind to make sure I have the best information needed to build the best life for myself and my family. Out of all the success-focused books that I've read, Perspective: Rewire Your Brain for Success and Abundance is one of my favorites. That's not just because of the information it contains, but also because Chris Boman takes such a unique and effective approach by combining clinical studies with hardcore science and his own experience; he then simplifies that information into one body of work we can all understand and use.

One thing this book isn't going to do is give you any quick fixes. In *Perspective*, Chris talks a lot about the importance of getting to the root cause of our problems and explains tactically why this is a better long-term approach. Chris's approach stood out to me right away, and I think it's a real strength of this book. We all need to be thinking long-term about ways in which finding a root cause can change our lives. Again and again, I hear people say, Yeah, but what can I do right now? I need to fix this problem NOW. But that's not how it usually works. Instead, we all must figure out what is causing the problem before we can start to see real solutions and growth. Only then can we really start thinking of long-term sustainable health, whether that's going to the chiropractor once a week, eating healthier, or embracing a new exercise program.

The reality is that most of us need a real change in perspective right now. So many people focus on instant pleasure and have no sense of how today affects tomorrow. They don't focus on their health until it's too late: they wait until their backs are against the wall before they actually focus on improving their body, going to the chiropractor, or thinking about what they eat or whether they exercise. *Perspective* helps you think through these topics and more. It provides practical tools so you can take care of your body before you start feeling stressed or lethargic—before your body begins breaking down. Personally, these are issues of paramount importance for me. Health is such an important part of my life, and I believe it should be for you, too. Don't believe me? Imagine you've built the perfect business. You have millions of dollars and all the time and freedom in the world, but you also have poor health and lack sufficient energy to get through the day. That almost defeats the entire purpose of what you worked for.

Our personal health is more than just the opportunity to enjoy our business successes, however. It's also the most important step in becoming truly successful: good health is the foundation of fulfillment, happiness, energy, peace of mind, and wellness. Not nearly enough Americans focus on its importance. The United States is number one in the world for obesity. The rise in different types of diseases in the world means a new perspective on our health is essential. A lot of people give me the excuse that they're just going to live their life until it's "their time to go." That kind of thinking doesn't work for me, and it shouldn't work for you. What if you could extend your time with your loved ones and the people you care most about? What if you could have more energy with your kids as they grow up? If you took just a little bit more of a focus on your health versus a day-in-the-life moment, think about how much longer and richer that life could be.

That's the kind of long-term thinking Chris Boman espouses. He does so by focusing on a core message that advocates freedom and abundance, two concepts I deeply value as well. A few years ago, my organization, Game Changers Academy, conducted a study. We asked 2000 successful entrepreneurs about their business goals. The answers we got were varied: some said they wanted more clients or a better business. But when we asked those same entrepreneurs what their larger end goal was, almost 90 percent of them told us that they want to invest in themselves and their families so that they have the freedom to do what they want with the people they most care about. What that tells me is that almost everyone's end goal is freedom. None of us want to believe that we are born so that other people can tell us what time to show up to work and what to do when we get there. As human beings, we like to have flexibility and variety; we want to be able to spend time with our kids, to travel, and to live life on our own terms.

I'm not going to lie: getting to that end goal by way of this book is an intense experience. There's a lot of information to digest here, and it's not a light, easy beach read. So take it one step at a time and realize that whenever you take on a big task and start to feel overwhelmed, it means you are growing as a human and expanding your capacity. That's a good thing. You're growing; you're learning more.

Finally, I'd be remiss if I didn't also say how great a person Chris is. Part of my career as a success coach involves speaking with people all over the world. I meet a lot of great ones, but I rarely build lasting relationships where I can become friends and really get involved in their lives and businesses. I'm glad to call Chris a friend. He has so much passion, vision, and drive. He's also one of the most genuine people I've ever met, and he truly has a deep desire to help people. He puts others first.

Chris and I first met when my wife went to see him as a patient at his practice, Trailhead Chiropractic. She returned feeling better than she had in a long time, and she insisted that I make an appointment as well. "He's amazing," she said. "It's a great practice, a great culture, and there is just so much good energy there." I told her we already had a chiropractor and didn't need another one. But she insisted, and eventually, I agreed to try him out. Chris and I hit it off immediately. His energy and his passion were contagious, and it was clear to me that he always goes the extra mile for the babies, children, and pregnant women who come to see him. Eventually, Chris joined my academy and became involved in our business development programs. There, I saw the same dedication and passion Chris brings to his practice. He's a forward thinker, and he's not afraid to go against the grain or reject traditional approaches. He sees that the economy is changing, and he is adapting and pivoting fast. Chris is someone who constantly invests in himself and bets on himself. Anyone who bets on themselves and puts people first is someone I want to be friends with, and their mission is one that I also want to be a part of.

I've been a successful entrepreneur and business owner for over a decade. I'm always looking for competitive advantages and a way to cut through the noise. When I find a book that amplifies what is important, that shows how to turn a vision into reality, and that places an emphasis on health, I know I've found a massive competitive advantage. Perspective does all of that and more. You could watch a dozen YouTube videos, or you could buy twenty-five business success books, and you still wouldn't get the valuable, practical information found here. So if you are someone who values your time, if you value your family, if you value freedom and abundance, the best thing you can do is read this book.

INTRODUCTION

HAVE YOU EXPERIENCED A MOMENT OR SEASON IN YOUR LIFE when you hit rock bottom and confronted failure face-to-face? You felt your heart go heavy, your stomach curl, and your tongue go dry as you contemplated what went wrong and what you were going to do next. As that moment became a season, food began to taste stale, and you found yourself looking for any distraction from reality. You couldn't sleep at night because you were stressed out about payroll or simply paying rent. Your alarm went off morning after morning, but there was zero motivation to get out of bed. You were, or maybe even still are, stuck with wondering: *Will I ever be successful?*

I get it. And believe me: I've been there.

I hit my own rock bottom in the fall of 2019. I'd been working as a chiropractor for almost five years and was experiencing rapid growth each season. I decided to hire an associate chiropractor, and, to quickly fill her schedule, I splurged on a very expensive marketing program. Up to that point in my career, I had been very specific about my target market for patients (I focus on prenatal care and helping kids with special needs). But I wanted to make sure I kept my new associate busy and that I had enough business to pay her salary. As a result, I threw to the wind my targeted approach and decided to grow my practice as fast and furiously as I could, marketing my services to anyone with a spine, including the coupon hunters and window shoppers. New patients and free consultations started streaming in—as many as twenty or thirty a week—but few of them stayed for long because I was advertising one thing, but in reality, selling them another. These new patients wanted a quick fix, and I wanted to help them get to the root cause of their issues. Between all of the initial paperwork and the diagnostics required to provide good chiropractic care, I was literally spending hours getting a new patient situated, only to have them basically reject my recommendations and then walk out the door again, never to return. All of that intake work also meant I had to funnel to my associate more and more of my established patients who loved me, and consequently, even they were beginning to feel like things at Trailhead Family Chiropractic were changing.

Despite my marketing and delegation efforts, my practice was falling apart, and I needed to start making some budget cuts. I turned off the expensive marketing program, and, predictably, the new patient stream dried up. I began noticing bigger and bigger gaps in my schedule because I had lost a lot of my established patient base as well. I had to email my accounting team to lower my paycheck each week to make sure everyone else got paid, and eventually, I had to lay off most of my staff, including my associate chiropractor. Here I was, thinking I was poised for exponential growth, and instead, I was watching my patients and bank account decrease dramatically each week. My wife and I were down to our last $300 in our checking account, and I was looking at failure face-to-face. I didn't have enough money to pay my receptionist, let alone give her the raise I had promised, and I was at the point where I was willing to sell my practice and let the entrepreneur dream fade away. I woke up each morning with zero motivation, and I ended each work day frustrated that nothing had changed and wondering if anything ever would. I couldn't see a way out of this hole I'd dug for myself: in other words, I was at my rock bottom.

Out of desperation, I decided that the only way I would be able to keep going was to apply for a $30,000 business loan that I knew was only a bandage for my real problem. I knew that this loan would only make things worse in the long run, but the decision was fueled by my state of stress and desire for temporary relief.

My perspective was near-sighted and, instead of trying to defuse the bomb going off, I was choosing to deal with the aftermath of the explosion. But, the Lord works in my life in funny ways. When the damage was reaching its peak, I was scheduled to go on vacation. So not only did I have no money, but I didn't even have the opportunity to earn any.

While on vacation, I sat at the dining room table, bags under my eyes from the lack of sleep, filling out the online loan application when my wife, Jessica, walked in and asked what I was doing. I sheepishly admitted to her that unless I got this money now, there wouldn't be a next payroll. "I have no choice," I told her.

Jessica was skeptical. Our faith has always been important to us, and she asked me if I'd prayed about this decision before committing to it. I hadn't. When I told her as much, I felt convicted and frustrated but reluctantly closed my laptop. I didn't see the point, but I trusted that she had a different perspective that I desperately needed.

I've seen countless people go through struggles similar to mine. For some, they go through this process multiple times, and the failure takes much longer than a few weeks to overcome. As a chiropractor, I also see this in my practice daily: some adults come in with chronic and debilitating health issues, kids struggle with simply learning to talk, and babies suffer from colic so bad their parents have to pay a babysitter just to get a couple hours of sleep. I have talked with business owners who are ready to throw in the towel just like I was. They are scared, desperate, and confused as to why things didn't work out. Again and again, they tell me they've tried every possible solution, and none of them seem to work. "That's okay," I always tell them. "*We got this.*"

THIS IS DIFFERENT

When I closed that laptop on vacation, it meant more than just refusing to get a loan. It meant that I was free to be myself again without worrying about making money (simply because there was nothing more I could do). A week went by, and we ended up having enough for payroll. This process of having just enough happened for about a month, and at that point, I was scheduled to attend a local chiropractic seminar. It was there that I started to remember why I chose chiropractic in the first place. I decided to rededicate my practice and career to my original mission and purpose and chase my big vision once again. That next week was different, and things started clicking in my mind. I realized that the real reason new patients stopped booking and that established patients left was because I wasn't living a life congruent with my core values: instead, I was seeing patients for all the wrong reasons. I was so interested in growing my patient base and making money that I dismissed why I became a chiropractor to begin with. I'd lost my perspective and was working for what I could selfishly get out of life instead of how I could provide value to those around me. I was living in scarcity instead of in abundance.

Once I realized how I fell to my rock bottom, it became easy to climb out. "Easy" doesn't mean it wasn't hard; it meant I was able to live my natural self. I returned to memorizing my patient's' names, taking an interest in their lives, and focusing on their well-being beyond just the adjustment, rather than what that adjustment meant for my bank account. That change alone meant that I was immediately happier, and so were my patients. They began referring friends and family members again; my schedule filled up organically, and I began to receive invitations to give workshops and lectures around our community again. I'd reconnected with my purpose by remembering my why, and, as a result, everything else in my life began to shift into place. More than that, I'd moved from a state of stress to one of abundance. I could once again dream and craft a vision beyond making weekly payroll. Moving into 2020, a disastrous year for most, we enjoyed financial security. My family and I began to take more vacations, and I was also able to buy my dream car (which I will talk more about later) cash-up-front and begin to build our family homestead. A shift in perspective was all I needed because success was already in me, and abundance was waiting for me to ask for it.

Perspective: Rewire Your Brain for Success and Abundance is a playbook for anyone who wants to find their perspective shift in order to live their very best life and experience success and abundance as my family and I enjoy. In the following chapters, I'll combine neuroscience and health tips to help you first create a physiological and neurological state of ease. You will also learn how to find your selfless purpose, core values, and selfish why. Additionally, I'll teach you how to craft a vision and set goals to live a life in pursuit of it. I will also give you insights on the skills I learned in order to ask the right problem-solving questions and how to develop and maintain the abundance mindset you need to help you climb out of your rock bottom and create the life of your dreams. Reading the book is the easy part; however, the tough piece is actually implementing what you learn, but that's okay. Together, *we got this.*

CHAPTER 1

THE PHYSIOLOGICAL PERSPECTIVE SHIFT

I TAKE SERIOUSLY THE TRUE MEANING OF DOCTOR (WHICH IS "teacher"), both in my practice and while writing this book. If you cast a big vision but aren't healthy enough to pursue it, that vision will stay a dream and never become a reality. Your family is counting on you. Your community is counting on you. The world needs you to become all that you were created to be, because you are here for a reason and a purpose. I don't want you to get to a point in your life where you regret the health choices you made out of convenience or ignorance.

My hope for this chapter is that it not only changes your life trajectory, but also influences the lives of the next generation because right now, the future looks sick. Over half of America suffers from a chronic disease, and over 70 percent of American deaths are from chronic disease. What pains me about these statistics is that almost every chronic disease is a lifestyle consequence. This means, either in ignorance or intentionally, we are choosing pleasure over health. Sugar addiction doesn't just affect you; instead, diabetes, heart disease, and other metabolic disorders are starting to influence our kids. Over 43 percent of kids are suffering from one of twenty various chronic diseases (such as asthma, obesity, ear infections, etc.). To understand why I am so passionate about people advocating for their own health rather than relying on medicine as a lifestyle, ponder this: we could pay to solve American homelessness and ensure every person in the world has access to clean water and enough food with the amount we spend on treating chronic disease in America. It's time to be your own health advocate, do your own research and experience better health not only for better performance, but also because future generations are counting on us to teach them how to live healthier lives.

THE NEUROSCIENCE BEHIND THE ABUNDANCE MINDSET

In a neurological state of stress, our bodies are hardwired to be most concerned about our own immediate survival. As a result, when we're in a state of stress, we tend only to think about ourselves and our immediate needs. When I was afraid I wouldn't make payroll, I didn't have the bandwidth to question whether or not I was providing value to the people around me. I also didn't have the brainpower to think about my purpose or care if I was living in it. Our neurology literally doesn't allow us to think about our futures in moments like that. That's why it is important for you to understand how your body works when it's in a state of stress and for you to develop strategies to stay in a state of ease.

I'm not trying to make you a neurologist, and I hope to explain just enough neurology to shed light on a traditionally complex, but nevertheless practical, aspect of everyday life. Emotions and our senses are simply chemicals and energy that the brain adds learned meaning to—just like sounds are just waves of energy. Our brain is responsible for making sense of all sorts of stimuli and telling our bodies how to adapt to them. I know this is sort of a primal way to look at humans, but understanding it is the first step to also understanding the neurology of decision-making, because the brain is processing a trillion bits of information per second (actually about a thousand trillion logical operations per second), so it needs to develop default operations to streamline your decision-making process.

The main one we'll focus on is your autonomic operations, which is the division of the nervous system in charge of automatic (subconscious) bodily activities, such as heart rate, breathing, digestion, hormone regulation, etc. While I don't like to just spew facts, here is what I want you to know: when a perceived threatening stimulus makes it to your brain, the amygdala, or fear center, is activated. The amygdala's job is to tell the rest of the body to run from or fight the perceived threat. Its only goal is to help you survive, regardless of where you run or how you fight; therefore, reactions that grow out of this stimulus tend to be a lot more impulsive, rather than thought-out decisions. The other way the amygdala is activated is if the brain falsely triggers it. This actually happens more commonly than you think, because the brain acts this way when it doesn't have all the information it needs to make a rational decision!

Think about walking around at night when you can't see anything. You are very cautious and are sensitive to every creak and knock you hear, ready to react at any moment. The body is very intelligent in that it knows its stress response will ensure short-term survival, so even when the body gets overloaded physically, chemically, or emotionally, it will cause something to happen in your spine called the subluxation. This is poor movement of the spinal vertebra resulting in a lack of sensory information to the brain, which ultimately causes the brain to trigger the amygdala's stress response.

I'm explaining this because if you continue to live in a state of stress, either due to real danger or through chronic subluxations, you'll be making decisions that only benefit you in the short term; both conscious and unconscious consequences happen as a result of your stress response. Think about your average salesperson. Their goal is to actually activate that amygdala by using tactics such as the fear of missing out: *The price will be higher tomorrow! Sale ends in one minute! Going fast! Limited supply!* These phrases are all designed to get you to buy impulsively because of the threat of not having that thing before someone else gets it.

But while these sophisticated responses have done a lot to keep our species alive, they also come with a cost. When we're triggered by a fight-or-flight situation, our body also triages all of our remaining bodily functions, focusing primarily on the ones most immediately related to our survival. In that state, the sympathetic nervous system (a division of the autonomic nervous system), which manages our stress response, can put a pause on activities in our reproductive system; it can also halt tissue repair and even digestion. You can start to see why long-term sympathetic dominance can cause high levels of inflammation and, in turn, be the root cause of many chronic symptoms.

I see the result of this fight-or-flight mechanism manifest in my patients in a variety of ways. When we are stressed, our brain makes decisions based on what it thinks is going to most immediately protect us, rather than what is rational and in our best long-term interests. It compromises our ability to form accurate memories; it alters our perception of risk; it encourages us to fall back on habits and prejudices, rather than exercising situational awareness and critical thinking. But all of these impulses, which are so helpful when we find ourselves in a life-or-death situation, can be really damaging when we're contemplating big life decisions like beginning a new career, entering a relationship, buying that new car, or eating in an unhealthy way. Instead of focusing on the big picture, our brain focuses on the picture pixel by pixel. So step one to creating a physiological perspective shift is getting into a neurological state of ease.

Chiropractic care is one thing that will help you deal with the stress perpetuating subluxation. Using sophisticated technology (we talk about this later) and well-trained hands, chiropractors detect and correct the spinal subluxation, thus allowing the body to revert back to its natural state of ease. This state of ease allows the body to heal and perform to its optimal potential; thus, chiropractic is good for everybody, no matter the symptoms you are trying to overcome. While chiropractic, in my opinion, is one of the most critical lifestyle habits used, there are many other things I want to share that you can use immediately to shift your neurological state and reduce your inflammation.

THE 3 TS

I hope you just learned a ton about your nervous system and why seeing a chiropractor is so important for you and your family's health routine. In this section, I am going to teach you how to further reduce your neurological stress with other lifestyle hacks. Chiropractic can help unravel the stress in your body from the subluxation, but we also want to ask, "Where do the subluxations come from?" In this section, we will dive into what chiropractors refer to as the "3 Ts" of stress, including trauma, toxins, and thoughts (or emotions). Even if you have a medical background, this will be a ton of information, and it is designed to introduce a new health paradigm to you.

When your body becomes overwhelmed with stress in even one of the above categories, that stress could be the catalyst that triggers your brain to activate the fight-or-flight response. This response causes tight muscles, especially along the spine, and over time causes subluxation, which, as you learned above, perpetuates the fight-or-flight response even longer and sometimes in more intense ways. The goal of a *chiropractic lifestyle* is to minimize or even eradicate these responses. I will use this term, *chiropractic lifestyle*, many times in this book, and it describes a person whose health habits include chiropractic adjustments, a positive mental attitude and life outlook, a diverse and nutrient-dense diet, and consistent physical exercise. The goal of this lifestyle is to reduce chronic stress (thus inflammation) and increase overall adaptability. A highly adaptable person is capable of more strenuous and challenging tasks and is usually known for creating world-changing value and solving the most challenging of problems.

Let's dive into the 3 Ts and learn more about how the everyday person can see life through the lens of a chiropractor and enjoy the benefits of living in the chiropractic lifestyle and cultivate world-changing adaptability.

Physical Life Traumas

We will classify physical traumas into micro and macro challenges. I am going to be as precise and action-oriented as possible, so get ready to implement.

Micro traumas include things like: repetitive behaviors, too much sitting, incomplete recovery from injury, and overall, not enough healthy movement. Most people don't even realize that having their computer screen tilted slightly to the left will create long-term problems such as arthritis, joint scarring, and muscle imbalances. Studies show that if a joint has reduced mobility for as little as four weeks, scar tissue begins to build up. This is a defense mechanism to stabilize an increasingly unstable joint. This change then causes the joints above and below to overcompensate, which leads to overuse. Over time, the cartilage wears down, bones start to touch and reach out to each other to fuse and permanently stabilize the joint. I believe the body is intelligent, so while arthritis and natural joint fusions are inconvenient and painful, it's much better than continual joint dislocation!

To overcome and prevent this cascade of events is to have healthy movement routines every day (arthritis doesn't have a rest day) and to properly recover from injuries. If you are sitting all the time, swap out your chair for an exercise ball or bar stool throughout the day and buy a platform that allows you to shift from sitting to standing and back. Make sure your computer screen is directly in front of you rather than to the side. If repetitive movements are your nemesis (grocery check stands, golf, etc.) try moving through the opposite range of motion periodically throughout the day to try and keep your muscles balanced and activated. Recognize that if you are doing the same thing over and over for more than a few hours at a time, it is always recommended to recover! Most people think only professional athletes need massages, cryotherapy, healthy diets, and the like, but if you are even a truck driver or tractor operator, you should be recovering at the end of your day by stretching and ideally enjoying routine massages and chiropractic care.

Macro traumas are major events such as car accidents, broken bones, or other serious injuries that usually require medical attention. So many times, as a chiropractor, I encounter people who will want to treat only until the symptoms are gone, when really it takes months of work to actually heal! It is always recommended to use an integrative approach with different therapists and doctors who work on a specific aspect of recovery (muscles, joints, cellular, emotional, etc.). While it would be impossible to be comprehensive, here are a few things that people might not think about when recovering from a major injury.

After most surgeries, I recommend starting physical therapy as soon as possible to prevent muscle atrophy. You should pay attention to not only strengthening the muscles, but also restoring the neurological pathways that have been disturbed due to the fight-or-flight stress response. The brain will naturally want to protect the area long after the pain is gone, but it is important to put the brain at ease and use the full range of motion of the joints or muscles in the area. In conjunction, I recommend cellular therapies such as infrared light, PEMF, cryo, and lymphatic drainage therapies. Finally, there is also a myriad of mental healing methods, some by chiropractors that use the NET technique, and others by therapists that use the EMDR technique. During your healing with therapists, you will also want to make sure you are consuming a healthy diet centered on reducing inflammation in the body, which is what we will touch on next.

Chemical Traumas

As I was with physical traumas, I will be to the point when discussing chemical traumas, as I can talk about this subject forever. If you haven't really followed your nutrition closely, this will be like drinking water from a fire hose, so if you feel overwhelmed, you are not alone. Every time I finish this section in a lecture, I take a strategic water break so everyone can digest (pun intended) all the information.

When we are talking about chemical traumas, we are really talking about everything from what we eat to the literal chemicals in our environment, and that is how I will break up this section. Again, I want to make sure the perspective you have when reading this is that this information will help stop the fight-or-flight cycle, putting you in a state of ease, and thus allowing you to dream big and create big visions for your life.

In my opinion, what you consume either contributes to health or disease. Not everything you eat will immediately give you a disease, as your body should have enough adaptability to detox the occasional dessert or fast food. Disease happens when environmental hazards find a hospitable environment in the body. Even though the medical profession at-large is dependent on medications to alter body chemistry, they are still resistant to people claiming to prevent and cure disease by changing what enters their body. I sympathize with them, in that there is an endless amount of snake oils and false advertisements claiming that one specific product cures everything. While a product might be a game changer for one person, it will never be a cure-all, because everyone's chemistry is different and thus needs different things. A prime example of this is our newly founded garden on our property. For years we have tried to grow our own food, but time and time again, the plant just shrivels up and dies. This year, my wife found a specific natural fertilizer that has been a game changer. Now, despite our super hot days, our garden is a lush green paradise. We figured out that our well water is alkaline, and so our plants need more nitrogen than the average garden on city water. This nitrogen allows the plant to be in balance and adapt to the outside stressors. The nitrogen doesn't cure the plant; it just provides a solution to a deficiency the plant needed to better adapt to the hot sun and soil ecosystem. Like a plant, many people may find that a probiotic could be healing for one person, just as going gluten free or adding vitamin D might be for another. In any of these cases, the supplement or regimen itself isn't the solution, and it won't have the same effect on everybody.

The point I am trying to make is that as I go through various chemical toxins and alternative suggestions, you still have to be in tune with your body and figure out the messages your symptoms are trying to communicate. No one knows your body like you do, and most doctors work on averages, not personalized solutions. I am not saying a medical doctor can't help—because I have great relationships with many doctors—but your health is ultimately up to you, and with Google in your pocket or purse, the only excuse I accept is, "I don't know what questions to even ask Google to start finding out the answers I need," and that is what this section is about. I hope to bring things to your attention that previously might not have ever been on your radar so you can become an expert in what you need to do for a healthy brain and body.

FOODS

You have heard the saying "you are what you eat," but I like to take it one step further and say "you are what you eat ate." This means if your lettuce processed chemical Miracle-Gro, guess what you are processing? If your plant absorbed Roundup, guess what you are absorbing? If the steer that became your hamburger ate sprayed and genetically modified corn, again, guess what your body is processing. Living in Southern California, I have incredible access to organic, non-GMO food, but I know many states don't have that privilege. This is why I am an advocate for growing your own food as much as possible, but there are also many online options that ship less-processed options right to your door.

Let's first focus on animal sources of food. Our modern farming practices are so far beyond natural and traditional ranching and farming techniques that we have had to engineer solutions to problems we created, such as the need for massive machinery, sewage ditches, medications, food dyes, and so on. People have been consuming meat, poultry, eggs, and dairy for centuries, but only recently (and really only in the USA) are people starting to have allergies and reactions to these foods. In my opinion, it isn't the food itself that is responsible for these reactions; it's how the food was raised. Dairy cows live on overcrowded, bacteria-infested farms and are fed high-sugar grains. They produce an unnatural amount of milk and live well below a cow's expected lifetime. There are some farms that practice drilling holes in one of the stomachs of the cow and periodically "vent" the bloat caused by the grains and swap contents with another cow to share bacteria diversity to prevent disease. Our meat cows have been genetically selected to grow at astronomical weights and fed unnatural foods, and still some farms treat with antibiotics and hormones for growth and to compensate for an unhealthy environment. Traditional poultry farms, and even some labeled "cage free," cram chickens into small, smelly coops, where they are given a foot-by-foot "door" to go out on the little pad of concrete in the sun outside of their cage. Again, they are fed pesticide-ridden feed, sometimes treated with probiotics, and get so fat that they get to a point where they can't even walk, let alone reproduce.

Because of these farming practices, processing machinery has been sterilized, pasteurized, and essentially destroyed every good colony of helpful bacteria, making room for the bad ones to proliferate and cause problems. This is why there is a growing movement of regenerative farming and many outlets to buy "regen" products at your local farmers market or online markets. On my little family farm, we have a cow living on pasture eating a various assortment of grasses, clovers, legumes, and flowers, and drinking healthy, clean well water. We move her every day or two to a new patch of grass (as she would grazing in the wild) so she doesn't sleep and eat over her own manure. We milk her by hand, thus getting a bacterial exchange, and we drink her milk safely raw and make cheeses and yogurts with all the healthy enzymes intact. No bloating or changes in stool for our family (which we usually experience with traditional dairy), and it tastes very different than store-bought dairy. After a few days of letting the pasture sit, we bring the chickens on the manured pasture to spread it around and eat the fly larvae, thus preventing too many flies and the smell. The chickens are eating bugs and grass in the sun all day, and they are also a part of bringing life back to the land. No medications or hormones, mass sickness, or destruction of land at our place, and we also like knowing that we are contributing to building a healthier environment. So when you go to the store for your proteins, know that you are what you eat ate, and support farmers practicing a lifestyle that improves the earth, rather than destroys it (and you).

Next, we will focus our attention on our fruits and vegetables. There has been massive awareness about GMOs (genetically modified organisms) in the past ten years or so, but I still find it sad that there is an "organic" and "non-organic" section at the store. Before the 1990s, there was one type of carrot, apple, strawberry, and so on, but now we have to make a choice. Are the higher prices worth it? You can find many resources online that give insights on which organic foods are worth it and which aren't, but the more important question is, "What is the soil like that the plants used to make their fruit?" Even organic produce from the store can be significantly less nutrient-dense than non-labeled produce from the farmers market or your own backyard. We are trained genetically to pick the most vibrantly colored produce, and big agriculture knows this and sees that the food that is picked before it is ripe will not have the same colors as vine-ripened produce. Most crops that are shipped are chemically "ripened" to have the appearance of being full of flavor and vitamins but are really just aesthetically pleasing. This is how, in my opinion, so many Americans can be nutrient deficient despite eating what appears to be a healthy diet. This is also why we are all almost forced to supplement in addition to a healthy diet. The last thing I would like to mention about fruits and veggies is that not all "superfoods" are good for every person. Some people might have sensitivities to compounds in kale (lucky people) or tomatoes or elderberries, so it is very important to know what your body likes and doesn't like. There are also many tests available to monitor your body's sensitivities, as these can change in seasons or as we age. Just because you have eaten something for thirty years doesn't mean your body will always like it.

ENVIRONMENTAL THREATS

While this whole chapter could be a book (and might be later on), this specific section is constantly changing and evolving, because we are just understanding the effects of some modern inventions and practices. Some things might resonate with you; some might not. But again, remember the objective is to present information to you that you might not have been aware of, thus giving you the opportunity to do more of your own research on the subject.

The first thing I want to highlight is environmental chemicals. There have been water tests all around the country, and they are finding pharmaceuticals, heavy metals, pesticides, and other harmful chemicals in wild rivers, snowpacks, and the water coming out of our faucets (think Flint, Michigan). Our bodies are made up of about 60 percent water, but our brains are about 73 percent water; thus, consuming water containing neurotoxins, antibiotics, and carcinogens is naturally going to affect our body and brain's ability to adapt and perform at its peak potential. These chemicals contribute to your toxic load as well as injected pharmaceuticals, phony petroleum-based supplements, and beauty products. In my opinion, this is why intermittent fasting is so beneficial in today's day and age, because it gives the body a chance to detox the ever-present toxic load building up. My advice to you is to be careful buying expensive but just as harmful "natural" products, just as you should be avoiding chemical-laden makeups, deodorants, soaps, perfumes, house cleaning products, and hair products.

Next, are things that we might not be able to see but are definitely affecting us. Our culture is obsessed with convenience, so the marketplace is flooded with smart devices and appliances. We are always carrying our phones and, for most employees, surrounded by computers and the internet. These electronic devices and satellites can, and have been, disrupting our biomagnetic fields. While we don't fully understand why or how, I know some of the illnesses and diseases medicine is treating with chemicals are caused by electromagnetic sensitivities. I noticed a huge difference in my sleep when I started to keep my phone at least five feet away from me while sleeping and turning off my Wi-Fi whenever

I am not using it. There is a wide array of EMF harmonizers that work (and just as many that don't), which make it easy for your body to adapt to the increasing demands of more powerful Wi-Fi, cell signals, and other technological advancements.

Along the same thread is the amount of light stimulus our eyes are forced to adapt to. From phones, to computers and TV screens, our eyes are processing light spectrums way beyond natural and are definitely contributing to many ocular disorders as well as emotional challenges from the over stimulus. A simple, yet effective, trick I always have active is the "blue light blocker" feature available on every device. This reduces the overload of harsh light reaching your eyes and has made a huge difference in my life from reduced eye strain and headaches caused by too much screen exposure. The goal would be less screen time, but to keep up with our modern lifestyle and jobs, this workaround has helped many people continue to work and grind without the "tech hangover" after. Finally, while we are on the topic of tech, "grounding" has been a huge breakthrough for helping reduce anxiety and inflammation levels. The earth has a certain magnetic field as well that is attractive to harmful free radicals that build up in our bodies through the above-mentioned modalities. By standing on grass or dirt barefoot, digging without gloves on, trimming trees, and so on, you contact the earth and thus release these free radicals from your body. In my opinion, this is why it is so refreshing for me and so many others to get into the wilderness, whether it's backpacking or camping with the kids. While there are many more environmental threats, and more being released every day, if you master this list, you will be healthier, much more adaptable, and have a mind ready to create and impact the world.

Emotional Traumas

This is probably the most neglected source of stress and the most overlooked by doctors around the world. The most prominent health challenge usually brought on by mental stress is multiple sclerosis. For instance, one day a high-performing C-suite employee working sixty- to seventy-hour work weeks is brought to their knees by fatigue, muscle weakness, and brain fog. After months of tests and a few doctors, they learn that for years their body has been working overtime and eventually caved in to the stress in the form of a full system shutdown. The only way to heal is to lower the stress input physically, chemically, and most importantly, emotionally. As a chiropractor, I see mental stress manifest in the form of shoulder pain, occasional back spasms, anxiety, hormonal issues, and metabolic challenges. Usually a care plan of adjustments will get great symptomatic resolution, but once a patient accumulates that mental stress again, the body reverts to its state of overwhelm, and the symptoms come right back. To help people illustrate and identify their emotional stress threshold, I use the concept of a "mental ecosystem."

As you learn more about me, you will find out I don't live the typical Southern California lifestyle. Sure, I have a sports car, but, as you know, I also run a small regenerative homestead (@firstfruitshomestead). As I learn what it means to grow healthy plants and animals, I have been able to tap deeper into the real reasons why conventional foods aren't growing the way they used to: the soil is sick. For years we have burned the soil with artificial fertilizers and sucked the diverse ecosystem dry with monoculture (growing one type of plant) farming. The more I learn what it means to grow adaptable, nutritious, and diverse crops, the more I see the connection between the soil ecosystem and our mental ecosystem.

As I was not trying to make you a neurologist before, I am not trying to make you a farmer now, but I think it is helpful to use something you can see to describe something you can't. When you see a plant wilting or turning brown, that is a symptom that the plant is deficient in something it needs to grow. A good farmer will recognize this and diagnose the problem to nurse the plant back to health. A clueless farmer will assume that the plant will bounce back and will only react when the plant has no leaves and is clearly on the brink of death. When it comes to our mental symptoms, most people are the clueless farmer. It's only when they have anxiety and headaches so bad that not even medications are relieving that they seek alternative help. They only perceive they are stressed when they are actually overwhelmed. By that time, it requires a significant amount of effort to recover, and sometimes there is even permanent damage. So how can you be a good farmer to your mental ecosystem? Be aware of things that can overwhelm you physically, chemically, and emotionally, and either prepare to handle it before the stress comes or properly recover after the stress passes by. For example, our garden was getting tortured by the hot desert sun, so we put up a shade cloth and now everything is thriving. We planted things in raised beds to avoid them being easy pickings for critters. We water with compost tea to provide an abundance of nutrients to the dry and worn-out soil we are trying to rehabilitate.

Some suggestions for cultivating a healthy mental ecosystem include taking mental breaks throughout the day and frequent vacations for recovery, figuring out what recharges and energizes you after a draining experience, setting boundaries to avoid pests from picking away or stunting your fresh ideas and aspirations, and taking time to meditate and "walk through" the garden of your mind to check on relationships, projects, to-do lists, and aspirations to make sure they are in balance. Don't try to hang on to things that need to die, because oftentimes that death allows for something newer, better, and stronger to rise up in its place. In my opinion, the hardest aspect of diagnosing the source of mental stress is that it can come from so many different angles including a poor diet, physical issues, or emotional threats. This is why we talk about living the chiropractic lifestyle, because each system is either built up or torn down by the others. You are an organism, which means you are a cluster of cells that make up organs, which in turn make up organ systems, which need other organ systems to help the organism adapt and thrive in the environment. It's usually never one thing, but oftentimes, in my clinical experience, the mental ecosystem is the one that is the most neglected and impacted by all sources of stress in life.

If most of this information was new to you, you might want to read through it a couple of times, because I packed years of research and clinical practice knowledge into just a few pages. If you are interested in expanding your knowledge on any of the above topics, follow me on social media, especially my practice page, because I am doing webinars and seminars all the time that go over new research and explore these topics in depth. If you rolled your eyes at some of it, recognize all I am trying to do is expose you to different aspects of health you might not have thought about and encourage you to research more to make the best decision for you and your family. I am confident that the biggest world changers you and I admire—and aspire to be one day—prioritize their health and are exploring every avenue that can improve their mental performance. As we shift gears in this book, always keep your health and neurological state top of mind, and work on those things just as hard as you work on your mindset, vision, purpose, core values, and goals.

CHAPTER 2

THE PURPOSE OF PURPOSE

LIFE HAS A FUNNY HABIT OF THROWING CURVEBALLS WHEN YOU least expect it, and in my opinion, this is the purpose of having a purpose. It's not just a fancy life tagline, but a true source of motivation for you that keeps you focused on what you were put on this earth to accomplish. During the 1918 flu pandemic, chiropractors were responsible for saving thousands of lives, but they were also arrested and imprisoned by the hundreds for practicing medicine without a license. The American Medical Association also created impossible "knowledge tests" for those seeking a chiropractic license, knowing full well that no one could correctly answer the questions posed by those tests. That same organization also created a "Committee on Quackery" intended to destroy the chiropractic profession. Multiple chiropractors were jailed for practicing our profession (the main charge against them was "practicing medicine without a license"). Part of the criticism against chiropractic may have been justified: in its earliest years, chiropractors advertised that they could cure anything. In my opinion, that was really just an issue of sloppy language more than anything else. Chiropractic had managed to relieve all kinds of distress, and it was because of those early practitioners that previously "incurable" individuals, some of whom had been committed to insane asylums, were able to get the help they needed.

Chiropractic doctors have never claimed to be practicing medicine; instead, we have always been committed to removing *subluxations*, which is just a fancy way of saying misalignments in the vertebra. The effect of that was to create a better sense of ease by reducing inflammation and getting to the root cause of people's problems. That's why chiropractors today often talk about what we do as affecting dis-ease, instead of disease.

It wasn't until 1987, when a U.S. District Judge found that the AMA had been deliberately targeting chiropractors in violation of anti-trust laws, that the AMA formally reversed its position on chiropractic. In the 102 years between the first recorded chiropractic adjustment in 1895 and the federal court decision, dedicated chiropractors risked their freedom to provide holistic healthcare to people in need. Why? It wasn't just because they could help people with back pain. It was because they knew that doing so was creating a new alternative to medical care and spreading a new idea on health and healing that could liberate the United States and the world from a lifestyle of dependence on medicine.

The purpose of purpose is to help you live with purpose beyond yourself. I want you to create and live your dream life, not live someone else's.

In this chapter, we're going to explore how you can reveal your own sense of purpose and its connection to something greater. I'll share some of what continues to drive me and how you can apply those stories in your search for your life purpose.

A SELFLESS PURPOSE

In my experience, the most motivating and inspirational purposes are the ones that reach beyond your immediate needs for survival and project to the future to create legacy impact, as we saw with the early chiropractors. A purpose isn't just about what you can accomplish; it's about contributing to a larger plan, like trying to better humanity or make the world a better place to live. Instead of having blinders on and only asking what's in it for you, the more your purpose is about how we can work together and build a network, the more you'll see the value in what it takes to get there and the more you will be able to accomplish. I really want you to dig in and take this seriously. When you think about the major figures throughout history who have really made a difference, almost all of them had roots in the greater good. And while we may differ on exactly what "greater good" means, we can probably agree that it's about wanting to make other people's lives better.

That's true for some of the most successful companies out there as well. If you look at Microsoft or Apple or Facebook, you'll see that they all have their own unique role in making our lives better, despite some of the negative things those companies may do. Microsoft wanted a personal computer in everybody's home. Apple wanted to streamline technology and make it easy for everyone to use. Facebook was built out of a desire to connect people around the world. For me, making others' lives better for generations to come using chiropractic care is my purpose and, as you read earlier, is what has led to my success even through hard times. My journey to become a pediatric and family wellness chiropractor, however, helped create the selfless purpose beyond just being a chiropractor for my own enjoyment.

I grew up loving sports and was extremely competitive. My dad always counseled me that the key to succeeding on the field was good situational awareness: that the more I was aware of my surroundings and what was happening in them, the more I would be able to anticipate my next successful move. Often, these reminders from my dad came when I was playing outfield on a little league team, where I usually spent my time daydreaming and looking at butterflies. Missing a few pop fly balls taught me that there were real consequences to my lack of awareness. That, along with a desire to please my dad, meant that I internalized his lessons pretty quickly.

As I grew up, my brain became highly trained to be aware of my surroundings on and off the field. On the soccer field, I learned to watch body language to see where opposing players were going to pass; in football, I knew who was getting the ball before the play even started. My growing awareness of my surroundings also meant that I was rarely caught off guard. I learned not to make rash decisions, which also meant that I could keep my cool and stay in a state of ease amongst chaos around me. That kind of level-headedness also meant that I could make strategic decisions that would help my team win.

By eighth grade, I'd decided that football was my favorite sport. I wasn't the biggest player on the team (in fact, I was pretty small by football standards), but I'd figured out how to be one of the smartest. I loved watching the sport as much as playing it, and I spent hours studying game tapes and reviewing plays. Along the way, I became even more adept at anticipating what the other players would be doing and how to be in the right place at the right time. Because I'd spent so much time practicing fundamentals, I could also make some show-stopping one-handed catches and terrific spins that ended up in highlight reels. In the world of my tiny Christian school flag football team, I was a star. I was certain I was destined for the NFL.

When it came time to go to high school, my parents decided to transfer me to public school. They thought I'd be safer making the transition to full-contact football at a larger school with a more experienced coaching staff. In that regard, it was definitely the right move. But even with the expertise of first-rate coaches, I struggled with the transition. For instance, I'd never even worn a helmet before, let alone thigh, hip, and shoulder pads. The first time I went for a catch, the ball bounced off my helmet; I literally had no idea how far the faceguard jutted out. When I ran, I looked like Mulan in that scene where Mushu instructs her to "Stand up straight, head high, and march!" With her arm and legs moving awkwardly throughout the camp, she was a spectacle (and embarrassment) to watch. So was I. I also struggled with the newly required skills of a full-contact game. Being tackled was not a ton of fun, of course, but learning to tackle was even harder: I'd explode forward toward the ball carrier, only to have him swat me away like a bug. It was all so humbling—and frankly, a little demoralizing. I quickly went from being one of the most confident members of a team to one of the most tentative.

As an athlete, I saw a chiropractor, and I spent a lot of time in the waiting room there with very little to do but read the magazines and look at the walls. The chiropractor just so happened to specialize in sports medicine, and his walls were decorated with signed photos of professional athletes. By this point in my life, I'd made peace with the fact that my biggest football achievement was going to be riding the bench of my school's varsity team. As for my professional football career, that was clearly never going to happen. Truth be told, I wasn't going to make it as a college football player, let alone a professional one. And if I wasn't going to succeed in that environment, I needed to find a new one where I could.

The posters and memorabilia on the chiropractor's wall gave me a new brand of situational awareness, particularly when it came to thinking about my career. I knew I loved the camaraderie of being a team player, and I knew I wanted to help people in the future. I also knew how hard it had been for my dad to work his way up the corporate ladder, leaving the house at 3:00 a.m. every morning so that he could avoid the worst of Southern California rush-hour traffic. Each and every workday, he drove three hours roundtrip, often returning home after the family had finished dinner. By the time he arrived home, he was tired and wanted to take it easy, or it was about time for us to go to bed. I knew I'd never survive that kind of lifestyle, and I didn't want to be forced into a job that paid well but didn't feel gratifying to me. I knew I didn't want to be told what to do; I wanted to make my own schedule, and I wanted to work close to home. I looked around that chiropractor's office and thought about *his* lifestyle: there were framed photographs of him hanging out with all these athletes I enjoyed watching on TV, pictures on the field, in the arena, and on the golf course, all showing that he was living life to the fullest doing what he loved. I thought about how much better my family member and I both felt after we were adjusted by him. It was clear our chiropractor loved what he did, and if his car and his vacation photos were any indication, he was definitely making a great salary. My high school guidance counselor had suggested that I consider physical therapy as a career, but I had no idea what physical therapists really did and why. At least from a patient's perspective, I understood chiropractic care.

I knew that if I specialized in sports chiropractic, I could parlay what I loved about football into an entire career that promoted holistic healthcare while also helping other athletes realize their dreams. Plus, I'd still be near the game, so I could continue to enjoy the camaraderie of a team and the excitement of a winning season.

The final decision to become a chiropractor happened when my teacher asked us to write a paper on a career we were interested in. I got the opportunity to talk to my chiropractor about his profession, and that conversation cemented it in my mind. From that day forward, I told anyone who would listen that I was going to become the best sports chiropractor in the world. I enrolled in every advanced science class offered at my high school, and I made sure that I actually studied and understood the material, rather than just cramming the night before, because I knew I would need the information later. When my guidance counselor asked me what I wanted to major in, I had no reply. I literally told him I wanted to be a chiropractor and showed him the classes I needed as prerequisites to start chiropractic school. We looked at the majors offered by the University of Montana (thank the Lord they actually had a major that fit), and I chose Exercise Science. Now, for this major I had to take one of the most rigorous classes offered at the university: Anatomy and Physiology with Lab. The teacher was known for failing people, and the course often caused students to even switch majors because of its difficulty. I had transferred in from community college on an academic scholarship and took the rest of my general education credits my sophomore year.

My junior year, however, was when I had to take the dreaded anatomy class. I also informed my counselor at the university that I had to take physics and organic chemistry for chiropractic school. She looked back at me like a deer in the headlights. She explained the top three most difficult classes at the university were anatomy, organic chemistry, and a literature class. I was proposing to take two of the three hardest classes at the same time. Oh, and my credit load for semester one was twenty-one credits and semester two was twenty-two (full time is considered twelve, in case it has been a while). This didn't phase me at all; in fact, I welcomed it, because I knew there were going to be semesters in chiropractic school that required thirty-plus credits. I had a bigger purpose than just getting my undergraduate degree. I was all-in pursuing my dream as a chiropractor, but in hindsight, this approach was probably risky; I was so focused on preparing for a doctor of chiropractic program that I didn't bother with courses in any other disciplines. That meant there was no plan B if I didn't get into chiropractic school, but once again, my purpose to help athletes perform their best and live a dream lifestyle gave me that tunnel vision I needed to focus and sacrifice partying, blowing off class, and settling for average grades.

I took so many credits at one time that I graduated with my bachelors a semester early and was accepted to my preferred program at Southern California University. I chose SCU because of its sports residency program, which was one of the best in the country (they regularly send their fellows to practice at the Olympics or to work for professional sports teams, two big dreams of mine). I was so focused on my ultimate purpose, that I didn't even attend my undergraduate graduation ceremony because I was already in my second semester of chiropractic school. By the time I enrolled, I was already fantasizing about traveling around the country with the Raiders and standing shoulder to shoulder with some of my favorite football stars during games. By the time my second year of chiropractic school rolled around, I was well on track to make that dream a reality.

As a chiropractic student, I was a seminar junkie and wanted to learn as much about the practice as I could. I knew I wanted to be the best, and the best didn't rest on weekends. One particular seminar during my second year in chiropractic school, however, changed the trajectory of my entire career and created my selfless purpose that would remain a part of my identity forever. It was at a workshop by renowned pediatric chiropractor Dr. Tony Ebel.

During his lecture, Dr. Tony described to the audience how he was helping kids with everything from autism and ADHD to depression, anxiety, epilepsy, and ear infections. I listened as he talked about how neurodevelopmental issues were becoming more pervasive in kids, and he described the very real ways he had seen chiropractic make those same kids lead better, happier lives. As he spoke, all I could think was, *Whoa. This is a game changer. Do other people know about this?*

And then Dr. Tony said something that shook me to my core and still gives me goosebumps today: "I can't imagine how frightening it must be for kids to be locked out of a world that they want to be a part of." That assertion literally knocked the wind out of me. Here I was wanting to selfishly help elite athletes continue to destroy their bodies for entertainment, when there were families out there desperate for help and answers that they weren't finding anywhere else. Professional athletes had already chosen their careers; I wanted to make sure kids like the ones Dr. Tony was describing would have the same opportunity.

From that moment forward, nothing mattered more to me than wanting to help each and every family who felt trapped by chronic health issues and the distress they caused. There was only one problem with this change: I knew next to nothing about babies and small children. I didn't grow up with younger cousins or even younger neighbors. As an adolescent, I'd never been a babysitter or a camp counselor, and I'm pretty sure I had never held a newborn. My understanding of a "blowout" was a hairstyle and "reflux" was the knee jerk from the doctor tapping the knee. I knew I needed to invest in some extra training, because this new, deeply rooted purpose was worth it. So not only did I start training with Dr. Tony Ebel's program, but I also started the path of becoming a diplomat of pediatric chiropractic. The internationally recognized organization ICPA trains thousands of chiropractors in every aspect of pediatric and prenatal chiropractic and offers a 400-hour postgraduate program that takes about one weekend a month for about two years. Even with all the book knowledge and the necessary training to be qualified to see these kids, I still didn't have a lot of hands-on experience with that client base. Needless to say, I was nervous, but my purpose burned deep in my heart and inspired me to change the lives of everyone who visited our office.

I was fortunate to have this laser focus from high school on what my purpose was supposed to be, but I know a lot of people aren't so fortunate. I want to tell you a story that reaffirmed for me that I was living within my purpose after graduating from chiropractic school. When you are living in your purpose, your body and mind unite and it seems as if the universe is compelling you to do something: when you feel slightly overwhelmed but know you have to press forward, when challenge excites you, and when you can't stop talking about something are all good signs that you are close to working in your purpose.

One of my most influential patients was an eight-month-old baby named Jeremy (name changed for privacy). He could barely move his head and was diagnosed with a condition called torticollis, which is when the muscles on one side of a baby's neck lock up. Beginning at just two weeks old, he had been prescribed physical therapy two times a week. When I met Jeremy, he had seen zero improvement despite the rigorous therapy. His pediatricians had gotten to the place where they were ready to perform surgery to cut the muscles in his neck, stretch them out, and reattach them.

Jeremy also had acid reflux so severe that he couldn't keep down milk or formula. He was constipated, often for a couple of weeks at a time. As far as his mother was concerned, I was their family's last hope.

Jeremy developed these conditions as the result of a traumatic birth experience. His head got stuck in the birth canal, so the doctors tried to vacuum extract him out four different times, during which Jeremy's heart rate plummeted and they resorted to doing an emergency C-section. They had to pull Jeremy back up through the birth canal and through the stomach using excessive amounts of force in his head and neck. This trauma to the upper neck stressed out his vagus nerve, which in turn stressed out the rest of his neck muscles and digestive system.

And so, even though I was only six months into my practice and I hadn't had much hands-on experience with babies, especially cases this severe, I knew exactly what to do. Something in me knew I had to help this baby, no matter what it took. Even though I was nervous and felt the weight of the responsibility of taking care of Jeremy, I leaned into the opportunity. My mind centered, as if it was in the eye of a storm, and my hands seemed to move instinctively. What happened next was actually pretty anti-climactic. I gently adjusted Jeremy, as it only takes the pressure you use to test the ripeness of a peach to perform the adjustment on his top vertebrae. Jeremy's mom looked at me like, "Great, my last hope touched my baby's neck and called it done. Who do I go to for help now?" Nevertheless, I told the mom, "Please go straight home as I expect (what I know now to be) a blowout." Again, I got the crazy eyes look back, but I assumed she did what I told her to. The next time I saw her, which was the next day, I could tell something dramatic had happened. I asked her what had happened, and she told me that I had been exactly right: he had a blowout. I knew with that response that we were on the right track: Jeremy had been living a life of intense stress, and now we had gotten him one step closer to living in a state of ease.

After the next adjustment, Jeremy started turning his head just a little bit. Little by little, his acid reflux started getting better (not the knee-jerk reaction, but the constant spit-up), and his mom could reduce the antacid medication he'd been taking. The next week we started noticing that his head was turning fully back and forth. A couple of days after that, we started noticing that Jeremy wanted to sit up. Then, he began crawling, first backward and eventually forward. It was a clear progression of improvement, and in just a few weeks we'd gone from a baby who was on track for a failure to thrive diagnosis, was scheduled for surgery, and was taking at least four different medications, to dramatically reducing those interventions and allowing him to meet developmental milestones. His mother was much happier, and I had affirmation that I was living in my purpose and that this was something I could do for the rest of my life.

Through chiropractic care, Jeremy was given the opportunity to live a relatively normal childhood, free from the dependence of medicine. In the intervening years, I have had the time to really think about the different ways my selfless purpose manifests in what I believe and what I do. I know now that, more than anything, I want to build a lasting legacy for each and every one of my patients so that they can go out and fulfill their own purpose in life. As my vision has grown, my purpose has expanded even further to helping people as a six-figure strategist for service-based businesses and helping you by writing this book (a mental adjustment). I am blessed and excited every day I get to help others find and live in their purpose because I believe that, through my work, humanity as a whole has a chance to experience life at its full potential. By reading this book, you are also helping me change the world.

That deeply rooted purpose is what wakes me up in the morning and helps me persevere through rough times. Experiencing yours will give you a new sense of drive, renewed energy and passion, and most importantly, a new reason to live. In the rest of this chapter, we'll talk more specifically about how to define and refine your purpose and also realize the core values that protect you from going too far off course as enticing, but purposeless, opportunities tempt you. These next few sections will help you troubleshoot and expedite a sometimes-long journey to truly realize and live in your purpose. As with the chapter before, this section is written with little fluff and as much practical information as possible. I also use some stories and illustrations that I feel help convey technical information as easily as possible.

RUNNING TOWARD SAFETY, RATHER THAN FROM DANGER

Just as my farming journey has taught me much about myself, my hunting adventures have had a similar effect. I feel like hunting is not only a great way to provide healthy meat for my family and see the wilderness off the beaten path, but it also exercises your ability to stay calm under extreme stress. When I can't be out in the wild hunting, I like to watch hunting shows on TV to learn new strategies. On one particular show, a group of guys were hunting antelope, which tend to graze in wide-open fields. The hunters didn't have the kind of tree cover they would if they were hunting other animals, so in order to get within range of the antelope, one of them used a decoy. Standing behind a vinyl cow, the hunter could slowly walk toward the antelope without startling the herd. The antelope may have thought the decoy looked or even smelled weird, but it was normal enough and moving slowly enough that the antelope decided it wasn't a threat until it was too late. By the time the herd realized they were in danger, one hunter had already pulled the trigger. The remaining antelope herd turned and ran the opposite way, not even concerned if they were jumping off a cliff, so long as they were running away from the immediate danger of the hunter. The herd had no idea where they were actually running to, let alone if it was in the direction of safety.

When we simply run away from a situation, we are making similarly impulsive, unexamined choices. Those antelope were so triggered by their flight instinct that they literally had the capacity for nothing other than just to get as far away as possible. Think, in contrast, how a meerkat slowly emerges from its hole, then quickly jumps back down and only comes out when he knows he is safe. Even if a hawk does threaten him, the meerkat knows exactly where his hole is as a retreat to actual safety.

So ask yourself: is your neurology allowing you to make long-term decisions out of a state of ease, or is your amygdala forcing you to simply run away from danger, but in no particular known direction? Oftentimes, this can be as simple as checking in with our bodies and minds, assessing our breathing and ability to concentrate, and noticing whether we're able to relax or feel agitated.

Another way is to ask yourself: *am I running to something, or am I running away from something?* If the answer is that you are running away, you're probably in a state of stress. Examples in my life include considering selling my business in 2019 so I wouldn't have to manage the stress of buying an incongruent marketing system hoping I could "get" a massive influx of patients. Examples in yours could include wanting a new job because you don't like yours, retail therapy, procrastination, lying, cheating, or simply causing trouble with other people to overcompensate for your own personal problems. It is helpful to examine the source of stress and to determine if you should be actually reacting with your fight or flight, or if it is simply a *perceived* threat that doesn't actually pose a real danger. If the threat is real (no new leads, kids won't obey, no money for rent, etc.) have a plan to activate that won't just get you away from the situation, but instead move you toward a solution that will help you solve the problem.

ROOT CAUSE ANALYSIS

Once you've identified a safety plan, it is important to figure out the root cause of the issue, so you don't react to just the symptoms of something deeper. So often, a new patient will arrive in my office frustrated and looking for an instant cure. They've been experiencing chronic lower back pain and are tired of taking handfuls of medications each day. Parents of my younger patients repeatedly tell me they've tried everything to help their child manage a neurodevelopmental disorder and that nothing has worked. The first thing I always say to everyone who walks through the doors of my practice is this: chiropractic care doesn't cure anything. Instead, chiropractors help you uncover the root cause of your symptoms and enable the body to function the way it is supposed to by removing the source of stress (the subluxation), which allows the body to heal itself. My job is not only to help you understand when you are living in stress and how to react in a healthy way, but also to diagnose why that stress response was triggered in the first place. Discovering the root cause behind the symptoms is the key to enjoying your body's optimal potential, whether that is breaking the record for the fastest marathon or being the best stay-at-home mom in the universe.

Let me give an example of how I help people who come into my office find the root cause behind their symptoms, then we will go over strategies on how you can apply them to your life. I begin every new patient appointment with an in-depth discussion of their health problems and their health goals. Then, as part of our state-of-the-art scientific testing, we use infrared thermography, surface electromyography (EMG), and posture analysis to find exactly where a body is expressing inflammation, muscle spasms, and overall stress. These tests allow me to see how effectively a patient's nervous system is processing and communicating neurological signals from the brain to the body and vice versa. We also include an in-depth discussion of a patient's problems to try to get a sense of the external stressors that may be complicating their overall health, including diet, exercise routine (or lack of one), and emotional factors like a toxic workplace or troubled relationships. Gathering all of these assessments can tell me a lot about how stressed their nervous system is and how that stress is manifesting in their body in the form of symptoms.

Looking at infrared thermography and surface EMG allows me to understand which levels of the spine are stressed out, which can also lead me to understand what organ systems are also working in a state of stress.

Indicators of stress from the test in the upper neck mean that there is severe stress at the base of the skull. That is the main area for parasympathetic stimulation (sorry, last bit of neurology) or relaxation to most of our organ systems including endocrine (hormones), digestive, heart, lungs, and so on. Someone that has stress in the upper cervical spine is typically struggling with things like headaches, stiff neck and shoulders, anxiety, depression, and problems sleeping, because the symptoms are all effects of stress in those organ systems.

In my pediatric cases, when I see stress at the top of the neck, typically a patient's complaints are colic, ear infections, and sleeping issues, because that's their manifestations of stress in those areas. If we saw a patient with a severe amount of stress in the lower back, those are typically the reasons for low back pain and sciatic pain. Those nerves also go to the digestive system, which is one reason why we saw constipation issues in Jeremy, and irritable bowel syndrome or even auto-immune issues in other patients.

By hearing an explanation of the reasons behind the symptoms, my patients get the opportunity to make a decision to either continue to cover up their symptoms with medications, or approach it in a holistic way by addressing the stress in their nervous system and other lifestyle factors.

Think back to Jeremy, that first patient who came to me with not just neck problems, but also digestive issues. When I looked at his scans, there was severe amounts of inflammation in the upper neck, and then the middle and the lower. We noticed over the course of time doing these scans that the stress was going away, and that ran parallel with the symptoms getting better.

As a chiropractor, I can't turn off my analyzing mind, so when I am out and about I am constantly noticing people's posture. If our bodies are in alignment, we stand with our hips directly over our heels, our shoulders over our hips, and our ears over our shoulders. Doing so allows us to maintain our center of gravity with the least possible amount of energy and strain. I can learn a lot about you based on any variation in that alignment, including your current emotional state. In fact, I used this skill to wow my then-girlfriend, now wife, on our third date. I told her that I could tell the demeanor of a person merely based on their posture. When she asked me to analyze her, I nailed her emotions perfectly.

This is also really helpful in shedding new light on why my patient is suffering from chronic problems. For example, if your hips are tilted backward, I know you suffer from tight hamstrings which, in turn, may be causing knee pain. A slumping posture may mean you have poor core strength, but it also may mean you're experiencing depression or fatigue. Jaw pain may actually be the result of stress building up in your neck and shoulders. This is my trained skill of *root cause analysis,* the art of seeing a symptom and identifying its root cause. I want to teach it to you, not to impress your next date (not recommended) but to get to the root cause of obstacles and problems that will come along the way. If you haven't done this before and get frustrated, it's okay. Like I mentioned, it is a skill that requires practice, failure, and dedication.

SO WHAT AND SO THAT

If you've ever spent any time around a kindergartner, you know that they are curiosity machines, always asking why. We lose that curiosity over time, due to increasingly stressful responsibilities that trigger our stress response. We also lose the ability to self-reflect and start relying on habit. We adopt a kind of blind herd mentality, which can have disastrous consequences. If we are going to get to the root cause, we have to be willing to look at all aspects of our lives differently. Think back to the antelope on that hunting show. If just one of them had been suspicious of the strange vinyl cow advancing toward them, they might have had a very different outcome. Instead of taking a few steps left or right to get a better view of the decoy and what might have been behind it, they just took a quick look head-on and decided everything was okay.

Humans do this all the time as well. We're constantly looking for the easy answer or the one that requires the least amount of thought. We avoid and resent the effort involved with the really hard questions. To find our true purpose, we must instead learn to embrace these hard things. We must begin to examine what is behind our perceptions and to question what we think we know. To do that, we also need to get back to that five-year-old self who was always asking *why*.

My strategy is to ask myself: *So what? And so that...*

When I wanted to open my own practice, I looked in the mirror and literally asked myself: *so what?* When I wanted to write a book, launch a startup, get married, and many other big decisions, I made sure I could answer that question truthfully and completely. The times I didn't ended up in disaster (cue fall of 2019). If the first answers of *so what* involve anybody else except you, keep exploring. If anyone else is involved in why you want to make a big decision, you most likely are NOT living or uncovering your purpose. Instead, you are literally being crop dusted behind somebody else's. I want you to remember that image you just had, along with the weird smell that just appeared out of nowhere when you discovered you are doing something aligned with somebody else's purpose and not your own. Get out from behind them, find your own lane immediately, and breathe the fresh air that comes with forging your own path. It's important to peel back the layers and figure out what's really motivating you. Without that information, you're never really going to know what you're aiming for.

The next phase is asking yourself *so that...?* Say a guy goes to a store to buy a drill bit. His true purpose wasn't to own a new drill bit. Instead, he bought the bit *so that* he could drill a hole. But he didn't buy the bit simply because he wanted a hole. Instead, he drilled a hole *so that* he could put an anchor into the wall. And he put the anchor into the wall *so that* he could install a bookshelf. He installed the bookshelf *so that* he could display books, and he displayed the books because it improved the look of his bedroom. That made his wife feel happier about their space, and she wanted to spend more time with him there. *That* is the real reason he bought the drill bit. And the bit itself was just a small part of everything else that he was actually doing.

Let's say you're not happy with your job. Maybe you feel under-appreciated and underpaid and overworked, so you want to do your own thing. But if we dig deeper, you might tell me that the real problem is that your job is cutting into too much of your time and energy, and you don't have anything to invest in other aspects of your life. Maybe you want to start your own business so that you can have more time to spend with your friends or family. You're investing in a new company, yes, but more than that you're investing in relationships so that you can enjoy a full life. You can have the energy to play with your kids or take your family on vacations and live a life that's not dependent on your work schedule. Instead, you can live in freedom and you can be there for your kids.

Or maybe you come to my office and tell me that you want to lose twenty pounds and get your blood pressure down. If I ask you why, you might say *so that* you can run a marathon. And if I ask you why you want to run 26.2 miles, you might say that it's always been a dream of yours because your mom used to run marathons and you want to attribute that memory to her and feel more connected in the process. That is the inspiration that will keep you going through the shin splints, ankle sprains, and running in the rain or heat, and will allow you to make it through Christmas without eating any of Aunt Karen's famous cheesecake.

I hope this was helpful in helping you ask different questions of yourself and your motivations and gets you started on the pathway to stepping into and living in your purpose. My final thoughts on your purpose conclude with your core values that help create "guardrails" to keep you on track.

Think back to when we discussed the importance of posture and think of your head as your purpose and your shoulders as your values. If they're not in line with one another, your neck is going to hurt, your jaw is going to lock up, and you're probably going to have a heck of a headache. If you tell me that you want to get your high blood pressure down to run a marathon and that you're still eating Big Macs for lunch, I'm going to tell you that your values are undermining your purpose. If you tell me you're eating organic food but you're washing it down with a bottle of chardonnay every night, I'm going to tell you the same thing. It's important to know what you want your life to look like but also have the conviction that every decision you make is either allowing you to grow closer to your purpose or is pushing you away.

DEVELOPING YOUR CORE VALUES

As I mentioned, once you've explored and understand your selfless purpose, your core values are going to act as guidelines to keep you on the path of walking toward and in that true purpose. I call this *value-based decision-making.* Here's another example from my own life about how this value-based decision-making works. I said earlier that I was so certain I wanted to be a chiropractor that I focused my coursework exclusively on that goal. I also made other value-based decisions around this goal.

When I was in college, I took extra courses instead of partying, and I decided not to drink because I knew if I got a DUI, I'd never be able to get my chiropractic license. I also made sure that I hung around people who wouldn't be in the middle of any kind of sexual assault or sexual harassment scandal; instead, I hung out with solid people where there'd never be a situation where I could be accused of that sort of thing. I put good food in my body because I valued it and wanted my body to function at its optimal potential. Don't get me wrong: I still ate cake at birthday parties and enjoyed myself, but I recognized that, in the long run, I was going to be able to make a much better difference if I started eating healthy instead of living on the typical college diet of McDonald's and Taco Bell, because I knew I wouldn't have the mental energy to take all of those classes and fulfill my goal of becoming a chiropractor. I promised myself I wouldn't even drink coffee until I graduated from school because I didn't want to become dependent on it. I also spent a lot of my free time shadowing successful chiropractors instead of just going out and doing whatever I wanted every weekend. I made sure I sacrificed time to network and develop professional relationships that have proved to be super helpful to me. These are just some of the examples of value-based decision-making in my own life. Sometimes it means sacrificing what you want to do for the sake of where you want to be.

You can determine some of the values you have unconsciously created by looking at some of your current habits. Do you say that you value your body, but you eat out at unhealthy restaurants four or five times a week? Do you say that you value your budget, but you still put toys and trips on a credit card you can't pay off? I made the decision to convert my practice to a cash-pay chiropractic office because, too often, I saw insurance-dependent patients who said they wanted to make a lifestyle change but never followed through. If your insurance is covering the bill, there is less motivation for you to really invest and care about the chiropractic lifestyle. But when people pay cash, it shows me and them that they value their health and believe they're worth the investment. Just the other day, a lady came into my office with her baby. She'd seen how beneficial our time with her daughter had been, and she told me that she wanted to experience for herself the same relaxation her baby was now experiencing.

We completed a full scan of her body, and the results were stress, stress, and more stress. It was clear she had never taken the opportunity to take care of herself and that she had been through a lot of trauma. I showed her the results and told her that her body needed some work (in the nicest way possible), but *we got this*. It was going to take time, repetition, and commitment to put her back together. I knew we could help and get her there, but it was going to take a real investment on her part. She told me her husband was never going to approve that kind of expense. I suggested she ask her husband what he values in the long run and where he is investing his money. She went home and pointed out that he had just purchased an expensive new bike and an Apple Watch he didn't really need. And then she asked if he really valued his toys over her ability to function with her family and be the best wife and mom she could be. In other words, she was able to use that as leverage to invest in herself and her care plan, because she and her husband both agreed that her health mattered more. It wasn't that they "didn't have the money," instead, they just had to choose between buying things that satisfied a want versus something that helped out a need.

One of the most obvious examples of value-based decision-making is our retired or retiring generation. A lot of people in my parents' generation have lived and worked primarily with the end goal of retirement at sixty-five. They've spent their lives making sacrifices and continually adding money to their 401(k). Their thinking is that it's worth making sacrifices now to save up a big nest egg so that they can really enjoy their retirement. Don't get me wrong: saving and investing is smart, but I'm not willing to sacrifice a lot of what brings me and my family joy along the way. I chose to find ways to make more money to pay for both. When Jess and I are on a date, if we feel like it, we'll order an appetizer and drinks. If we're still hungry after dinner, we'll get dessert. We will stay all nine innings of the baseball game rather than leave early to avoid traffic. I'll burn through the rubber on my BMW tires and buy new ones if it means an amazing day on the track. I don't want to sacrifice experiences I can have in my thirties for the hope of experiences in my sixties and seventies. I could make more money in my practice working by myself, but I would be sacrificing precious time with my family. I choose to employ a bigger staff because I value time with my family more than a padded bank account. One isn't right or wrong; you just have to decide what you value most. (The coronavirus pandemic has made this line of thinking very real for some people. Say you saved up your whole life to take a cruise, and now you're being told that you can't. If you value traveling now, you're going to be much happier if you figure out how to make it happen much sooner, rather than later.)

One way I make decisions is to make *value-based decisions*, which is to experience the most of what I value the most. The other is to create *core values* that act like truth serum in my decision-making process. The two main core values I focus on in my business and personal life are freedom and abundance. They influence and check all the decisions I make. For instance, most of the time my practice is overstaffed so that I can let a staff member take vacation time or extended family leave. That way, I know if someone needs time off or decides to take a new job, I'm not going to be scrambling to replace them right away because we have more than enough help. I employ two receptionists because that way, if one gets sick or wants to go on vacation, she knows she'll have the freedom to take the time she needs without worrying that the practice is depending on her. Those kinds of decisions allow everyone in my practice to work with that same sense of freedom and abundance. I also make a point of always paying people what they're really worth instead of making a decision based on a good deal. I could easily give my staff a flat bonus, and they'd probably be happy. But if they have earned a bigger one, it's important that I give them that so that they know how much I value them, and so that they have more freedom and abundance in their own lives. I'd rather sacrifice my own pay, because I'll live in abundance knowing that if I give them what they're worth, they're going to give me their all, even if it means I need them to work a weekend event or something else that wasn't on the schedule.

When determining your core values, once again you can ask yourself *why* before you make a decision. This time don't go for an end goal; try to uncover how that end goal makes you feel. Believe it or not, achieving goals isn't actually the only source of gratification. Everything you do can be gratifying and exciting (even paying down student loans) because you know it is a completely congruent decision based on your long-term goals, purpose, and core values.

If the prospect of identifying your core values leaves you confused and scratching your head, don't worry. There are a variety of exercises and thought experiments you can use to begin to identify them. One of the easiest is to journal everything you do for the next week. I do this with a food journal when I am trying to figure out someone's sensitivities. After that week you can reflect on why you did what you did and how you can orient your life better to reflect your true purpose. Whether we realize it or not, we all wear our values much like a Green Bay Packers fan wears green body paint and a cheesehead in negative-thirty-degree weather.

Once you learn to unpack those minute-by-minute choices, you can then evaluate them and decide if they truly support your stated purpose and bring real, long-term value as an asset, rather than something that will turn into a liability. Finally, once again remember, this is a skill. It's going to feel like learning to drive or riding a bike: very difficult at first and like there is too much to pay attention to. Break it down into little chunks and try one thing at a time until you can put it all together. Before you know it, you'll be joining me (and hopefully passing me) on the racetrack of life, pursuing your selfless purpose and in alignment with your core values.

CHAPTER 3

CASTING A VISION

Have you ever walked into a room and wondered why you were there? Often to help me remember, I retrace where I was to help determine what the overall goal was to begin with. Worse, have you stopped in the middle of your workday and asked, "What am I even doing here?" Or you look back on when you first got your job, thinking it was temporary until something better came along, yet here you are fifteen years later? Can you even picture what "something better" would look like? If not, that's a really good signal to you that you don't have a vision, and you're working in a state of stress to merely pay the bills.

A vision is a crucial part of living in your selfless purpose and living a life of success and abundance. One of my favorite examples that illustrates the importance of having a vision is the 1993 movie *Rudy*. In it, a high school student has dreams of playing football at the University of Notre Dame, but he doesn't have the grades to be accepted by the school or the athletic skills needed to play Division 1 sports. But Rudy is determined to live his dream, and he eventually enrolls at Notre Dame and decides to try out to become a walk-on player. An assistant coach realizes how driven Rudy is, and the coach offers to help train him. Rudy still faced unbelievable challenges, especially since he was so much smaller than the rest of the team. But those same teammates grew to admire Rudy's commitment, and after a new head coach refused to let him play, they all threatened to quit the team. The fans also wanted Rudy to play and began chanting his name during a big game. The coaches agreed to let him in for one final play in the game, and he managed to tackle the opposing team's quarterback in the process. The rest of the team carried him off the field on their shoulders in celebration.

One of the main reasons I love this movie is because Rudy wasn't just trying to make the football team; instead, he was doing it to show what can happen if you put your mind to it. If you work hard enough, if you believe in yourself, you can accomplish all kinds of things. Rudy wanted other people to be inspired to live out and pursue their dreams despite the obstacles. In terms of points earned or total number of sacks, Rudy didn't make that much of an impact on the team, but he made a huge difference when it came to the team's sense of comradery and their morale. He inspired the coaches and made his team work just as hard as he was. The fans cheered him on and lifted up everyone's spirits. And far more than just making a tackle, Rudy united the school and the community. That's the power of a vision.

In this chapter, I'll help you to explore a vision and explain why having one is so important for living a life of success and abundance. I'll also explain the cognitive dangers of being lost and what to do when you find yourself facing detours and roadblocks along the way. But first, I bet you're wondering, what exactly is a vision?

CRAFTING YOUR VISION

There's a poster hanging on my office wall that says, "My vision is that people would find chiropractic care before they say, 'I wish I would have found you sooner.'" In so many ways, that poster sums up why I do what I do in every aspect of my practice, from the actual adjustments, to how I treat my staff, to why I invest in marketing. It's not just so that I can make money or get dozens of new clients; instead, it's because I really believe the world will be a better place if more people embrace the chiropractic lifestyle. When I'm spending hours writing notes or I invest in a new marketing team, it's good to be reminded that those are steps toward a much bigger vision of making the world healthier. I can look at that vision and remind myself and everybody alongside me where we are going and why it matters. Having a vision requires you to think beyond your current abilities and resources. You don't have to know how it will come to reality, but it is important to be working toward something big. Goals, which we will talk about later, help you mark your progress along the way.

It is important for you to remember that we aren't always up on the podium, winning the award for all to see. Sometimes we're in the gym, trying to find the strength to get through that last set. You don't want to do it, and no one is watching you to make sure that you do. You know that you're going to be sore tomorrow. But you do it anyway, not just to show people you can win the next game or even the whole season, but to get better so you can make it to the next level.

Your vision will be different than mine, but a vision is never about your own accomplishments. When you cast a vision, you are inviting other people to join alongside you. When I ask clients to share their testimony about how their kids no longer get ear infections after getting adjusted, I don't do that to glorify them, and they don't agree because they want to glorify me. Instead, we do it together, recognizing that we are all coming together under the same vision, which is to make sure that moms hear about chiropractic care before their kids have gone through eight rounds of antibiotics and two rounds of painful tube surgeries.

As we talked about in Chapter 2, your purpose is fueled by your so what, so that questions. *Be a pediatric chiropractor; so what?* Because I want to make the world a better place so that my kids get to enjoy a life better than my own. Your vision, on the other hand, is furthered by your actions. To pursue my vision of making sure parents find chiropractic before saying, "I wish I would have found you sooner," I host workshops to tell. To tell the truth about chiropractic to the public, teach other chiropractors to be successful, and be a role model for those who could possibly make chiropractic their career. That involves being at my practice, marketing, teaching, writing, recording, networking, and so many other things as I work toward the world knowing about the impact and importance of perspective and chiropractic care. When you think about your own vision, remember that it's not just about you; it's about other people and accomplishing something bigger than yourself. That awareness is what will allow you to become a master visionary and to actually lead the people around you. In the rest of this chapter, we will talk about the downfalls of not having a big vision to pursue, and how to go about crafting your vision.

THE PROBLEM OF WALKING IN CIRCLES

Without a vision, it's easy to get lost. When we get lost, we tend to panic. Our behaviors as a result of that panic can vary; however, we all tend to become even further disoriented when we're in that state of stress. Hikers lost in the woods, for instance, will begin to walk in circles, even when they are certain they are still moving in a straight line. This happens because our brains are operating in a purely reactive state; we are looking for something familiar, or anything that will confirm we aren't as lost as we fear we might be.

As a result, our brains go into crisis mode. It's only when we can calm ourselves down enough to access the rational part of our brain that we can become proactive and actually begin analyzing our sensory information and making informed decisions. Instead of making ten bad decisions in a single minute, we begin taking ten minutes to make one thoughtful decision. What we previously thought was more time than we could spend becomes the most efficient way to get us home.

The problem with not knowing where you are going is that you're not going to be able to get very far before you make wrong turns or just start walking in circles. If you have to keep restarting over and over again or you have to turn around and go back, you are eventually going to fail to get to your destination, and you will have to start something new. I see a version of these patterns at my office every week. A few of my patients only come in when they are experiencing extreme pain or musculoskeletal distress. Because they've allowed their condition to deteriorate to that state, they end up spending a lot more money and time than patients who have embraced the chiropractic lifestyle and regularly come in for wellness visits or proactive assessments that can head off issues before they really develop. With the former group of patients, we have to be reactive and work backward to undo whatever is causing their suffering. On the other hand, the proactive patients are forward-looking and better able to anticipate—and prevent—the suffering coming their way.

That same process also works outside a chiropractic office. If you are an aspiring entrepreneur, you may have a goal of launching a real estate empire or maybe creating your own successful social marketing enterprise by selling essential oils or Monat beauty products. If you don't have a vision for where you want to take your downline organizational members, they are going to fall off the bandwagon and stop selling, which means you're also not going to succeed. I've had the opportunity to get to know people very high up in the essential oil business and other network marketing businesses, and I've seen that the most successful people there are the ones who are willing to mentor the people downstream. They are more than happy to share the secrets that make them successful and to help create customers for their downline people, because they know that helping that person will help everyone else as well. That includes figuring out how not to be annoying with your business. If those successful entrepreneurs had just started their businesses by recruiting people at their church or their Facebook friends, their organization would have fizzled out two months later. And if they had asked just their friends to become clients or to attend a product party, they might have seen a spike in sales for that one month because their friends felt obligated to help out and buy something, but they aren't going to have repeat customers because they didn't cast a vision for them. The next month, their revenue is going to go way down and they're probably going to lose friends. To be successful, you have to cast a vision and then sell it to them. That makes it a natural part of the process.

The fact is, if you don't know where you are going, no one is going to join you. It is incredibly frustrating to feel like you aren't actually working toward something. If you were one of those people who read the introduction to this chapter and realized that you've walked into a room and not known why you were there or stopped in the middle of your workday and wondered what you were doing, it could be because your boss hasn't cast a vision for you. Being an employee isn't inherently bad, and everyone can't be an entrepreneur. But if the leader isn't casting a vision, then it's hard to feel motivated about your work.

Just the other day, I realized how important it is for me to cast a vision so that my employees feel motivated as well. The husband of one of my employees recently accepted a job in Napa, and she came to me and asked if there was any way she could continue working for me remotely. I thought that was such a cool thing that she was proactive, because she values Trailhead and her work here so much that they almost didn't take the Napa job. I found a way for her to do her work remotely, and now we can continue to be a part of the same vision. Another employee of mine recently texted me on a Saturday night to say that one of the belts in her car had blown. Her back was up against the wall, and she offered to spend thirty dollars on an Uber to get to work, not because she was worried about her paycheck, but instead because she believes and recognizes how important it is for our office to provide quality care to our clients. She knows people are depending upon us, and she is so on our mission that she wasn't going to let anything stop her from doing her job. That's what happens when you have a business that is driven by purpose and vision.

If you're a parent, you've probably already become really good at this kind of vision casting. From the time we learn we're expecting a baby, most of us are already making plans for our children. We want them to excel at school and to have healthy social lives and creative outlets; many of us want them to pursue college degrees and meaningful careers. Preparing our kids for those eventualities doesn't start the night before freshman orientation at Harvard; instead, it is a process we begin either while our children are still in utero or shortly after they are born. The problems arise when we become so focused on one little detail or patch of ground (helicopter moms come to mind here) instead of familiarizing ourselves with the whole lay of the land, which in this case is our children's overall well-being.

I want you to realize this, because I know that setting a vision can seem intimidating. You may feel like you have to start from scratch after you have already worked hard to find your purpose. That doesn't have to be the case. Sometimes we already have a vision, but we just haven't made it very clear. Parenting is such a beautiful example of a way in which we obviously already have a vision, but we haven't necessarily made it clear. Defining that vision is going to be important because, whether you realize it or not, that vision is going to influence all of your interactions. When your kids ask, "Why can't I eat dessert whenever I want?" or, "Why do you discipline me?", the best answer is one that represents and explains your values. This is an opportunity to cast a vision that also lets them join you on that vision. For instance, you can say to your child who only wants dessert, "Well, your brain is important to me, and my goal is to help you be the smartest, most capable person. My vision for you is that when you eat your greens and your vegetables, you're going to be stronger, and the less sugar you eat, the better you are going to be." That invites your child to join you on your mission. (Will it work every time? No, but making it a habit will improve your chances!) You can also let them know that you exercise and eat well because you want to be the best daddy (or mommy) for them. This can help you reframe your parenting in very positive ways. Instead of disciplining your kids because your parents disciplined you a certain way, you have a reason, and that discipline becomes sustainable because you're doing it for the greater purpose.

Another thing to remember is that a vision cannot be born out of fear. Instead, it comes from being able to look ahead and think preventively. It's the equivalent of bringing your car in for routine maintenance instead of waiting for the check engine light to come on while you're driving down the highway. Not only does this keep you out of a scary situation (and a potentially expensive tow truck bill), but it also allows you to perform at your optimal potential.

Here in Southern California, where wildfires are common, we talk about that proactive mindset as *clearing the brush.* Rather than constantly fighting fires (a reactive posture), each season we weed out all the dead understory that might ignite and fuel a massive fire. Watch any group of backcountry firefighters at work, and you'll see them doing this on a much larger scale, often actually cutting lines of trees to create barriers the fires can't cross. Then, instead of dumping tons and tons of water on the inferno, they can systematically extinguish the fire by removing its source of fuel. Good forest managers will create a long-term plan for their acreage that includes selective cuts—and even controlled burns—to make sure they're not at risk for an uncontrollable disaster.

SEEING AROUND CORNERS

Several years ago, I was on my way back to my home in Los Angeles after visiting a girlfriend in Santa Barbara, which is about ninety miles north of the city. I wasn't familiar with the route, and I still didn't own a smartphone, so I borrowed my dad's old GPS for the trip. That particular day just so happened to be Super Bowl Sunday, so the already busy traffic on California's Highway 101 was worse than usual. Construction crews had installed a bunch of barriers and traffic cones, rerouting the already confusing flow of traffic. My dad's poor little GPS device couldn't keep up, and while I was waiting for it to tell me which freeway to merge onto, I chose the wrong off-ramp and found myself lost with a frozen GPS in the middle of the night.

Before I knew it, I was in a neighborhood filled with boarded-up buildings and lots of graffiti. The GPS was still stalled, so at the first marked intersection, I pulled over and called my friend in

Santa Barbara to see if she knew where I was. Turns out, I was in a particularly rough part of Compton, and by then, it was nearly midnight. I didn't want to get back onto the freeway, where I knew I'd continue driving in circles and probably end up in Mexico before I figured out where I was. I also knew the compass direction of my house, so I decided to take a chance and begin driving in that direction.

By that point, I was pretty worked up. I was definitely in an unfamiliar neighborhood and one that looked dangerous. My heart rate increased, I could feel the jolt of adrenaline in my bloodstream, and my palms became more than a little sweaty. As I continued to drive, my stress level increased, and I began making more and more unexamined decisions. Eventually, I saw the blue lights of police cars on the horizon. I had no idea if they were responding to a routine call or a serious crime. By the time I got close enough to realize they were manning a DUI checkpoint, I nearly whooped with relief. I got in line with the other cars and waited my turn. When a police officer finally approached my car, I explained the situation. He directed me toward Imperial Highway, a long stretch of road that cuts from Anaheim to LAX and that's marked by about a million stoplights. It would take me forever to get home that way, but at least I would know where I was the whole time.

As I waited at dozens and dozens of traffic lights that night, I had plenty of time to reflect on my reliance on technology. I'd put all my faith into that little device and, as a result, lost all situational awareness along the way. I relied on the GPS as my full source of information. I was at the mercy of reacting to the GPS instead of knowing what direction I should be heading. If, instead, I knew which general direction I needed to go and what general direction each freeway went, I could have at least known which freeway to choose. I may not have known the exact exits or streets, but I knew the major freeways and directions to keep me going.

When you are the only one who knows what you are doing and where you are going, you are going to get stuck, because you can only go so far by yourself and with your own resources. Even by just stopping to ask the cops for directions, I was inviting the police into my vision of wanting to get home safely, and they were able to contribute. Even though I had to go slower because of the stoplights, I was able to go much farther than if I had kept trying to accomplish my task on my own. There's an African saying I really love: "If you want to go fast, go alone. If you want to go far, go together."

Apps like Waze that promise the quickest way to get home from an airport or other landmark are even worse. When it comes to seeing the big picture, these apps actually do more harm than good, since they reroute us around traffic or construction and onto unfamiliar side streets. That can be great when we are running late and time really matters, but it also puts us in a place where we never really know where our next turn is or what lies around a corner. If your phone's battery dies or you lose cell reception along the way, you're going to find yourself totally lost and without any tools to reorient you.

When it comes to driving, there are some easy ways to avoid this problem, like taking a minute or two to preview the whole route before you begin driving or memorizing the main freeway changes and streets to look for. Always carrying a detailed and printed road atlas is another. These tips prepare you to anticipate multiple steps into the future. Just as importantly, they give you the tools you need to course correct if you get off on the wrong exit or miss your turn. To craft a vision and live a life of abundance, you must find a way to transfer this kind of big-picture thinking into other aspects of your life as well.

It can be difficult to think bigger when you are just starting out your business, so let me again fill you in on part of my story that you can use and modify to fit yours. I knew I wanted to run a big practice with multiple doctors from the moment I graduated. I wanted to do more than just go to work five days a week for the next forty years. I wanted to build a scalable and sellable business one day. This meant that, after starting in an environment with a staff that allowed me the freedom to build my practice with little overhead and established systems, I needed to rent a big enough space to grow when I moved into my own practice. I really only needed 1,000 square feet or less to run a profitable and busy practice, but I rented a space twice that big knowing that I wasn't going to use most of it until I had more doctors with me. As I mentioned before, I had more staff than I needed because I didn't want to bottleneck and stunt my growth. I never wanted to be too busy to see more new people. As we grew, I changed up my systems to prepare for problems that would occur with bigger staff or more patients, because I knew I was building something bigger than myself. I didn't know where I was going to find other doctors, and I didn't know if we would ever see enough people to fill the space, but now just three years later, I have another doctor and am continuing to grow while I spend more time with my family and pursue things that help me elevate my voice on a bigger scale. Seeing around corners is about anticipating needs before you need them and preparing for problems before they happen.

My clients tell me that they really benefit from having a notebook where they can write down the things they would like to accomplish or aspects of the world they would like to see change. Once you have a big picture, you can find your role in making it happen. People remember things much better when they write them down. Once you have that big picture clarified, post it somewhere you frequent to be constantly reminded and pushed to be better every day.

I know that many of you reading aren't just entrepreneurs, but family people as well. As I said earlier, parents are often masters of creating a vision, but they don't even know it. Most of the time the term "helicopter parent" is describing someone who is living in a state of stress without a vision for what they want their kid to learn. They try to stop things at every turn to prevent temporary pain or discomfort, thus disregarding the lifelong lesson they would have learned themselves. It is sometimes difficult to include your kids or let them do things you know are going to be problematic, but if you lead them properly and with vision, you can anticipate shortfalls and prepare for them so you both can still be growing closer to your vision together.

Let me give you a little example from our household routine that shows how this can work. My daughter Rosie loves making pancakes. On mornings when she and I are the first ones up, we like to make Mommy breakfast in bed. Rosie just turned five, which means she loves being part of making breakfast but still needs a lot of help in the kitchen. One of her favorite parts of making pancakes is cracking the eggs. She had gotten pretty good at it using store-bought eggs, but we just began raising our own chickens, and their eggs have much harder shells. The first morning Rosie went to crack one, she tapped the egg on the side of the bowl and then used her thumbs to separate the pieces, just like we had taught her. When that didn't work, she dug her thumbs in harder, which basically made the egg explode all over both of us and pretty much the entire kitchen.

The next time we made pancakes, Rosie again asked to crack the eggs. The exact same thing happened. So now we had a corner we needed to get around—I could just stop making pancakes with Rosie because the time it takes to clean up the egg aren't worth it, or I could find a solution that makes the process better. In the end, we compromised. I now crack the eggs, and Rosie mixes them into the batter. The vision is still to enjoy breakfast together and teach her how to be a little cook, but we learned to take a different route in order to stay on the same team.

Another morning routine that became frustrating was me being in the middle of making my pour-over coffee when Rosie wanted her vitamins. Now, each morning I place one on a counter she can reach, rather than having to stop in the middle of making my morning coffee. Just a little bit of forethought on my part prevented a lot of future frustration in our house and made sure that we all started our days with a smile. We can do the same types of things in our businesses, such as setting up email reminders, automated systems that can eliminate human error, and thorough training to avoid any elementary work problems.

This kind of predictive mindset is crucial to meeting your goals and pursuing a vision efficiently and effectively. Successful investors are good at their jobs because they have learned how to anticipate stock market changes and trends by looking at economic indicators. We can apply their techniques to our own entrepreneurship as well. In my career as a chiropractic entrepreneur, the challenge is to find new patients without being a salesperson, and also to convey the uniqueness of our practice and philosophy. One way I used to do that was to invest in advertising for health workshops, often purchasing expensive ads on platforms like Facebook to get the word out about an upcoming event. Early on, I could spend as little as $200 advertising an event to draw in fifty or sixty people. But as Facebook's algorithms changed, I found myself spending more and more money to reach fewer and fewer people.

The key was to develop a work-around in a proactive way, rather than scrambling to save an undersubscribed event the night before or to fill a week's appointments on a Monday morning after the Facebook advertising bottom fell out entirely. I began studying the effectiveness of social media influencer campaigns and how they might work in my industry. Not only did that change how I approach my work, but I also now offer programs that teach other chiropractors how they can leverage influencer attention in their own practices without spending a single dime on costly and potentially ineffective ad campaigns. Meanwhile, everyone involved wins: The influencers are receiving holistic healthcare, and they are sharing that experience with their tribes. Instead of spending money on advertising and risking a campaign that seems sales-y or inauthentic, the chiropractors are getting authentic endorsements with widespread reach. I always knew I wanted a busy practice, and Instagram barely existed when I graduated school, but now I am using it to accomplish goals and draw nearer to my vision.

Whatever your vision is, you want to remove little frustrations and anticipate adversity so that you don't get stunted in your growth. Most of the time pursuing a vision happens in stages, where you can't accomplish part B without completing part A. If your aim is to lose weight or reach a fitness milestone like your first marathon, get rid of every possible corner and anticipate the needs that are going to make it harder for you to exercise. If possible, dedicate yourself to a constant, non-negotiable workout time. If time is an issue, avoid mid-day workouts that will require you to shower or redo your hair and makeup before returning to work. When I was in school and working part-time jobs, I knew that even an extra minute of hassle would prevent me from getting a workout. Going home to change clothes was out of the question. Some days, even popping into a locker room to change felt like too much. In the end, I began weightlifting in the khaki pants and sports shirt that composed our uniform at the smoothie shop. I definitely wasn't going to appear on the cover of a fitness magazine with that look, and half the time I was covered in strawberry syrup and waffle cone crumbs, but I made the workouts happen and I felt a lot better for it. Oftentimes to accomplish something big, you need to do a lot of little things first that eventually add up to success. Without those workouts in college, I wouldn't have the strength today to see high volume and adjust without getting injured. Those little things and the choices I made contributed to the vision I am still pursuing six years later.

INEVITABLE ROADBLOCKS

We talked a lot about anticipating future needs based on your growth into your vision, but there are definitely times when unexpected things happen that you just have to adapt to. We call those roadblocks because they aren't just a wrong turn; they are a road's end. They're that burst water main on a major road that floods the street and forces us off our routes. They're the construction projects, avalanches, or washouts we literally never saw coming. If we're lucky, road crews are already on the scene, putting up barriers and detour signs, along with helpful police officers or construction workers with flags to get us around the obstacle and back on track.

But that's not always the case. Here's a story from my past about a literal roadblock I never saw coming. Back when we were looking at colleges, a friend and I took a road trip. We were both from Southern California, and I hadn't been out of the state much. As a high school senior, I knew I wanted to go to school somewhere rugged and wild, and the University of Montana seemed just the place. I applied sight-unseen, but when the acceptance letter arrived, my parents and I agreed it'd be a good idea for me to actually visit the campus before I decided to attend. So my friend and I loaded up my SUV and decided to take the backroads on what we were sure would be an epic adventure. This was 2009, before most people had smartphones. So, instead, we printed off pages and pages of maps and directions, along with every step that would get us the 1,200 miles to Missoula, Montana. The whole trip was going great until somewhere late at night in rural Idaho, where we drove up to a ROAD CLOSED sign. Neither my friend nor I had any idea what to do. Our printed maps only followed the route we had picked, and they weren't detailed enough to tell us about other roads. Besides, even if we'd had the best atlas in the world, it probably wouldn't have been able to tell us what to do. To make matters worse, it had been miles since we had passed a farm or a store. I called my dad and asked him to see if he could use the home computer to figure out where we were—and where we should go.

My friend and I both waited impatiently for my dad's old desktop to boot up. Once it did, the news wasn't good; as far as my dad could tell, the only work-around would require us to backtrack forty-five miles and then go at least as far out of our way again. My friend and I didn't much like the idea of wasting what would probably be two hours. As we sat weighing our options, an old Buick sedan pulled up alongside us. We felt like we were watching a Hollywood movie when the driver rolled down his window, let out a big cloud of smoke, and showed his weathered face. "You guys trying to get through here?" he asked. We said we were. "Follow me," he continued. "I'll go slow."

And so we were off, speeding down a narrow gravel road that was really more of a double-track dirt bike trail than any kind of road. Even with the SUV's all-wheel drive, I could barely keep up through all the dust as I watched the sedan zigzag left and right. I knew that if my friend and I lost our guide that we wouldn't have any idea where we were. But, miraculously, fifteen minutes later, we were back on the main highway—and back on our printed maps. I stopped to thank the driver, but he disappeared before I could. From that moment onward, I always thought of that driver as my smoking angel.

Barricades to our goals can be like that ROAD CLOSED sign in the middle of nowhere, Idaho. With corners, a lot of times we can see around them; however, roadblocks are those unexpected problems that stop us in our tracks. They can throw us totally off our game, without a sense of direction or how to problem-solve a new route.

The COVID crisis is a great example of this. Companies shelled out hundreds of thousands of dollars on marketing campaigns that became irrelevant when the coronavirus pandemic happened. Restaurants had ordered big inventories of food and made sure all of their positions were filled. Then suddenly, a week later, they had no use for the food and no shifts for their employees. It wasn't because of a bad purpose or a lack of casting a vision; it was just that they encountered a really big roadblock. We can cast a great vision, but if conditions change, we have to be willing to adapt that vision to meet whatever new realities come our way. In the case of the restaurants, their vision remains the same (keep their businesses afloat), but now they have to do things differently.

Roadblocks are important to understand because, when unexpected things come up, it can be tempting to throw away your vision and think that you did something wrong. Instead, you just need to figure out another way to get there. It might not be the same way you thought you'd get there in the beginning, but you still can find a way to get there, so long as you are adaptable in how you set your goals.

Say your goal is to run a marathon. Everything can be going as great as that college road trip was, until you accidentally break your foot, leaving you in an uncomfortable orthopedic boot or, even worse, a cast. Now, you're not only unable to log those training runs or trips to the gym, but your whole body is out of kilter thanks to that boot. Your hips have been thrown off balance, you're experiencing lower back pain, you're grumpy, and your sleep schedule is off. You can't make the broken foot go away; all you can do is re-route to get to your vision. To do that, you need your own smoking angel. And, even then, let's be real here: there is no magical dirt road that's just going to let you loop around a broken foot, but you can continue to work on your cardio and upper body strength. You can use a TENS unit to slow the muscle atrophy in your calf and do extra rehab sessions to get back on track quicker. You can also use some of that downtime to study running dynamics and learn how the successful marathoners rose to fame. In time, you can try swimming or some pool running to keep up your cardiovascular stamina. Eventually, you will heal, but all that time in the pool might have actually awoken in you an interest in an even more exciting sport, and competing in an Ironman Triathlon is your new, even more exciting goal.

Of course, it's still true that the more confident we feel in our ability to reach our goals, the more those roadblocks can derail us. For instance, as a chiropractor, I pride myself on a well-aligned and optimally functioning physical body. So when I wake up with back pain (and trust me, it happens to all of us), I feel particularly frustrated, since I'm literally supposed to be a walking billboard for a pain-free life.

Oftentimes, the only way to solve these roadblocks is to ask for help. When I was beginning my own practice, I learned invaluable lessons from mentors and professors. Some of my patients have become valuable consultants and collaborators. I wouldn't be where I am today if they hadn't been there to help me along the way. The idea of going solo, particularly in a big business venture or even a fitness goal, is paralyzing for good reason: being alone in the wilderness is as exhausting as it can be terrifying.

Let's go back to where we began this chapter, and that was with the idea of casting a vision that serves others. I mentioned in the introduction to this book that faith is very important to me and my family. A person in the Bible that illustrates the concept of "preparing the way" is John the Baptist. He preached about the coming of Jesus so that when Jesus entered the scene, people were ready to hear His message. I sincerely believe that God prepares the way for the big purposes he has laid within all of our hearts, and maybe roadblocks are designed to lift your eyes to something you would have completely missed. These roadblocks are not a time to give in, but sometimes they are an opportunity to explore other avenues to fulfilling your vision, and it's God's way of communicating to you in a way that you will hear Him.

As we move forward from roadblocks, I want to now talk just a little bit more about stress you most likely will be dealing with when a roadblock comes your way.

Eustress vs. You, Stressed

Remember in Chapter 1 when I was talking about the effects of stress? I was actually only telling you half of the story. The rest of it might really surprise you, because while stress can be the root cause of a lot of problems people are experiencing, it isn't always bad.

There are actually two categories for stress. The first is *distress*, which is what I felt when I got lost in Compton. But another kind of stress can actually be beneficial. If you've ever gone zip lining or skydiving or even just hiked a gnarly ridgeline, you've probably experienced *eustress*, or beneficial stress (the prefix *eu-* is Greek for good). Because eustress typically only lasts a short time—and often in a controlled situation—the chemical reactions it causes in our brains can be beneficial. An experience like a roller coaster ride or getting hooked into that monster fish can stir up stress, but it also leaves us feeling excited, more alert, and capable of increased concentration and performance, at least in the short term. One of my favorite sources for eustress is backcountry camping. Setting up camp, building and maintaining a fire, and being on the lookout for potential predators all create a little low-level stress, but they also make me feel super aware of my surroundings and survival in a very positive way.

I point out the important benefits of eustress here because we live in an era and a culture that loves to get rid of any variables possible. Most kids today where I live don't have the opportunity to ride their bikes around town and build forts all day. Many adults my age have forgotten the lessons they learned as the last generation of children who were really allowed to roam and experiment.

Minimizing risk is great, but don't throw the baby out with the bathwater. There is still a place for controlled risk in our lives. Whether it's taking a rock climbing course or getting out of your comfort zone long enough to sing karaoke in front of a new girlfriend and her friends, a little good stress can help us grow in positive ways and give us a healthy injection of adrenaline that reminds us we're alive and dynamic, feeling individuals.

The trick, of course, is to know the difference between *distress* and *eustress*. Weightlifting, for instance, builds mass by creating and repairing tiny tears in our muscles. That's a physical version of eustress. But lift too much too fast, and you may well create a much more serious tear, and one that could leave you sidelined for weeks.

Just as pressure makes diamonds, eustress can force something out of you that you might never thought of if you weren't put under a certain amount of stress. It's why most world records are broken in competition rather than alone, because the people around them make the athlete push harder. The stress of COVID caused me to look at other marketing opportunities that turned into another revenue stream. The stress of finding out my wife was pregnant and we were going to become a single-income family pressed me to work harder and build my practice faster. The short lesson here is there are times to lean into stress, and there are times when it becomes too much and harmful. Refer back to the first chapter when we talked about emotional stress to help figure out where that line is for you.

CHAPTER 4

GOAL SETTING

IF YOU HAVE A BACKGROUND IN BUSINESS OR ENTREPRENEUR-ship, you know that launching a new venture can be scary. When I graduated from chiropractic school, I knew that more than 20 percent of all new businesses fail within the first year or two, and that nearly half of these businesses fail within five years, including doctors' offices and wellness clinics. In fact, on my orientation day at chiropractic school they literally said most of you will fail school and most of those that make it will never pass boards, and most of those that start their own practice won't even be in practice in five years. What a first day, right? I knew I couldn't let myself become that statistic, so goals were a big part of my success and ability to beat the odds time and time again.

At the recommendation of my mentors, I offered special screenings and workshops to meet the community and to find new clients. It was a grueling schedule that kept me away from home most evenings, but I eventually began to build a base of regular patients. I started setting ambitious business goals for myself, both in terms of new patients and overall office revenue. Early on, I crushed each and every one of those goals, so I'd set even more ambitious ones for the next month. For instance, if I hit my goal of seeing forty new patients for the month of November, I'd commit to fifty new patients in December. At one point, setting goals was too easy, and I felt like even though I was hitting them I wasn't actually challenging myself.

There were times, however, when I stopped hitting my goals, no matter how hard my team and I worked. We'd write detailed monthly plans and schedule extra marketing events or spend more advertising money, but nothing seemed to make a difference. It was super frustrating, particularly at the end of the month, when we'd realize we had fallen short of our goals again. As time went on, I could sense that my staff was beginning to doubt me and my leadership, and that in turn made me question my own merit as a chiropractor, a business owner, and a CEO.

A few days later, I was on the phone with a good friend of mine, Tom of Roots Family Chiropractic in Chicago, complaining about my situation. I had missed my monthly revenue goal by $500; I'd fallen one or two short of my new client goal, and I'd missed my overall patient visit goal by about ten. I was pissed and ranted about my predicament. I could hear my friend start to laugh on the other end of the line, which only made me feel like more of a failure. I told him as much, and that just made him laugh harder. "Chris," he said to me, "you acquired forty-eight new patients in a single month, and you still feel like a failure? Why? Because you only met 99 percent of your goal?"

His observation was exactly what I needed to hear in that moment. I'd been so focused on those two missing patients I had forgotten all about the forty-eight I had brought into Trailhead. I'd also forgotten that December is a holiday month, when most people are more focused on visiting family or taking vacations than they are making healthcare appointments. Finally, I had failed to recognize that growth of any sort is rarely linear. Instead, it follows organic, sometimes circular, patterns. Charted over time, you see more reliable trends that every business person is looking for, but the day-to-day lived reality rarely follows that kind of tidy pattern.

In short, I was setting goals in a way that made sense to other people, but just didn't work for me. I was upset, my staff was frustrated, and I was getting burnt out trying to make this roller-coaster ride go in a straight line.

This realization really hit home for me when I attended yet another chiropractic seminar hosted by one of my mentors, Dr. Dave Jackson. He asked folks in the audience to list some of their recent wins. The responses had little to do with new cars they had purchased or income records, but instead, they talked about how they helped a patient avoid a dangerous surgery or how another patient had become pregnant after believing for years that she was infertile. They talked about saving lives and making people happy and would only occasionally—almost as an afterthought, really—add that they had broken their record for new patients or revenue earned. In fact, one of the guys on stage that weekend talked about how badly that kind of drive for new patients had served him. He had set a goal to see ten times the national average chiropractic office. He worked as hard as he could, spending weekends and late nights marketing and, eventually, he had come within 20 percent of his goal. Finally, he made it to his goal. As he was telling this story on stage, what really struck me was what he said happened next for him: after that Friday when he finally hit that magic number, he returned to work Monday, and guess what happened...*absolutely nothing.* There was no parade, no award or trophy waiting for him. In fact, no one else cared that he had hit that goal.

Hearing his story was a really humbling experience for me. I'd been setting number goals like his, thinking that there would be some big payoff in the end. I realized that there was never going to be a Super Bowl ring or even a giant bonus waiting for me, and setting high goals like that wasn't necessarily a bad thing, I just had no reason to go that high other than to be busier than other offices. Listening to that room of my peers, I began to realize that they were setting goals to create a lifestyle that they wanted to live (they did also have "selfish whys," which is a concept that I will dive into further into this chapter). I began to realize that many of the goals I had set were totally arbitrary. What, other than professional reputation and the thought that "the busier the better," was the reason for even having goals? Nothing, really.

I returned home not only with a much-needed new perspective that embraced my selfless purpose, but also excited to create my selfish why. I realized that when it came to goal setting, I had been doing it the way other people told me to, but it just wasn't working. At one point I did give up setting goals altogether to clear my mind. Doing that for too long, however, was a recipe for burnout because I couldn't see or reflect on my progress or have much of a direction moving forward. I knew I needed to pioneer a new way, because I couldn't be the only one that was struggling with goal setting and rewards. In the rest of this chapter, I will introduce you to that new way, which I call PAR goals, as well as your selfish why.

"SMART" ISN'T FOR EVERYONE

If my story rings true to you or reminds you of some of your own failed goals, don't worry: there's a good reason why. Most coaching and self-improvement programs are focused on what the industry refers to as SMART goal setting, which is creating goals that are:

✓ Specific

✓ Measurable

✓ Achievable

✓ Realistic

✓ Timely

There's a lot to be said for this kind of approach: we all want goals that are easy to define and not only attainable, but also easily tracked and evaluated. The problem with focusing on a SMART goal approach, however, is that it can quickly become an all-or-nothing focus. Also, this approach doesn't take into account all of the variables and curveballs we face along the way.

Instead, if we focus on goals that are *personal, attainable,* and *rewarding,* we'll be doing a much better job of setting ourselves up for success.

Let's go back to that disastrous fall of 2019 when I was certain I'd failed myself and my employees. I'd already set myself up for mental failure when I set linear goals month after month, despite various changes in workdays, holidays, promotions, and other month-to-month changes. I had no reason to focus on those numbers, other than that they were higher than the previous months. Also, they didn't really mean anything to me personally and had no real significance other than that they let me know my business was growing. That was never going to resonate with me in a meaningful way. Most importantly, those goals were never going to be rewarding in terms of advancing my vision, resonating with my purpose, and keeping within my core values.

Today, I'm proud that Trailhead Family Chiropractic is well on its way to becoming an elite pediatric and family wellness practice, but that's not because I'm looking to pocket more money so I can buy a fleet of fancy boats or a second, third, or fourth house. Instead, I'm proud of that status because it shows I'm providing massive value. That value is also reflected in my selfish why, but first let's talk about the system of goal setting.

ACHIEVING P.A.R.

In the world of golf, most athletes probably don't practice trying to get a hole-in-one on every hole. Don't get me wrong, every golfer would take a hole-in-one, but most of them aim for consistency more than anything. They practice the shots they can hit 99 percent of the time, rather than the magical shot across the pond, over the sand, and through the trees they might make once a year. The average number of strokes it takes for a golfer to sink a ball at any given hole (also known as *par*) can seem a lot less fancy than a hole-in-one. But if you were to make par on every hole every time—or even most holes—you'd be one of the best golfers in the world. Likewise, if you can consistently achieve goals that are *personal, attainable,* and *rewarding,* you're going to be well on your way to not only making your vision a reality, but also living a life of success and abundance.

Personal

Let's start with the personal. As I mentioned before, I am a chiropractic seminar junkie. A seminar I attend every year is put on by Dr. Dave Jackson. A lot of times, he begins this seminar by asking young, driven professionals this question: "If money and time weren't limiting factors, what would you most want right now?" Participants that haven't been through the exercise before say the classic "I've made it" symbols such as a personal jet, Lamborghini, or a fancy mansion on the beach.

When Dr. Dave pushes them further and asks why something like a personal jet is the goal they've set for themselves, their answers are also similar: they say that that's what they see "successful" people have and a way of establishing authority. Few of them even think to mention reasons like the time saved by avoiding the lines at commercial airports or inconvenient layovers and waiting for luggage to arrive. None of them say they're excited about airplane maintenance and hangar fees, not to mention the headache of finding and employing a qualified crew. For all of these reasons, a personal jet is probably the wrong goal for those seminar participants. It's definitely not one they chose for personal reasons. Only after Dr. Dave grills them on the reasons behind this goal do participants realize they're just giving answers based on societal expectations, rather than their actual values.

This is why I like to introduce the "selfish why." I know this might be different from the popular opinion of "your why," and I am not disregarding the power of family or personal tragedy being a powerful motivator. It's also not the *only* reason why you work or achieve your goals because, remember, your goals are attached to your purpose and led by your vision. The ultimate reason you do anything is for the betterment of the world for generations to come. We solve problems so that others can benefit and society can advance. Deeply engrained inside the human genes, however, are primal questions that must be occasionally answered: *What is in it for me? Why sacrifice so much? Why risk so much? Why not just settle?*

I know some of you have red flags going up because we have been so trained to believe that answering these questions is bad and goes against everything I have talked about earlier about adding value. I would agree with you if those were the *only* questions you are asking. Just like eating mayonnaise by itself is pretty gross, when combined with a hamburger bun or sandwich bread it makes the meal much more delicious. A selfish why by itself is not the only reason why you do what you do; it must be connected to a vision and a purpose. I'll give you an example. As I have mentioned before, I drive my dream car, a manual transmission

2015 BMW M3 tuned to just about 500 horsepower. It is a big selfish why for me, because when I get to drive home at 8:30 at night after a long day of seeing patients and teaching a wellness workshop, I think, *The sacrifice was worth it. This is awesome.* When I get to take my wife out on date night and drive through downtown, I have a big smile on my face because it's my time to bask in my selfish why. I don't work hard and help lots of people so that I can have luxuries; I have this luxury to motivate me to continue to serve and work hard, to remind me that the work is worth it, and that the rewards for me exceed the sacrifice.

I hope this was clear, and I am excited to see the smile on your face as you enjoy your selfish why as a side effect of the massive value you bring to the world. In the next section, we will talk about setting goals that are actually possible, then we will dive deeper into brainstorming rewards for your goals that can also be part of your selfish why.

Attainable

For a goal to be an effective one, it also has to be attainable. If you are a 5' 10" woman and you tell me you want to weigh one hundred pounds, that may technically be attainable, but it's going to be a struggle, if not just totally unhealthy. Our bodies lose weight because one of two things happens: either we increase the number of calories burned (mostly through exercise) or decrease the number of calories consumed (diet). Don't yell at me, I know there is a difference between healthy and unhealthy calories, but in case you forgot, we talked about that in Chapter 1. Are you really willing to limit your caloric intake below what we know is healthy for a functioning body? Are you willing to miss out on important life events because you're trying to squeeze in one more workout?

Determining which goals are attainable is one of the most difficult parts of this process and often requires the most skill. I realized this firsthand when I was setting financial goals early in my practice. I set a goal of, say, $30,000 a month in revenue, and then arbitrarily set a patient visit goal of 150 patients a week. What I wasn't doing was the basic math. In chiropractic, there's a statistic called *office visit average,* which is the real amount collected each visit when calculating variables such as discounts, add-ons, new patient fees, etc. I didn't know my OVA, which made it impossible to project how many patients I needed to see in order to hit that revenue goal. Every goal has an OVA, although it might look different for you than it does in a chiropractic office.

Let's say you're working as a landscaper, but you don't like your boss and aren't happy with the company, and you dream of starting your own landscaping business. You decide to quit your job and set December 31 as your last day. It may initially feel good to know that you've made that decision, but unless you've also calculated how many clients you are going to need and how many contracts to take or properties that you must have, you may find yourself in a financial crisis. To make this goal attainable, you must first do the math to figure out how many clients you are going to need, what you are going to charge, and what you will actually collect, of course accounting for the variables. If you are new to your business, you can either ask other business owners in similar fields or lay out your fee structure and reverse engineer. The simpler the fee structure, the easier it is to calculate how much you will actually be collecting per customer. If you are considering starting a stay-at-home business selling essential oils online to make enough money to quit your day job, you'll need to start by figuring out how much you will need per month. For ease of numbers, let's say you will need $1,000 per month profit. That means you need to sell $1,000 *plus expenses*. This means you have to think beyond just making $1,000. The most powerful punches come from the person who is focused on punching through you, rather than stopping at you. You have to have this same mentality when trying to hit your goals. We will go into detail later about how you actually hit your first dollar, but this section is focused on the mindset and overall strategy you need to win at goal setting.

Next, you need a plan that is scalable. Another benefit of seeing through the goal is that you can anticipate how to pivot when you get there. At some point in the essential oil business, you will change hats from a primary salesperson to a mentor of your downline. This means you teach other people to sell like you do, and instead of making impact one-to-one, you will do so one-to-infinity.

When you start a new business, you often don't have predictable metrics. One month, you might have ten new patients, and another month you may have none. Attainable goals aren't going to be linear ones from month to month. Here's another example to illustrate that. Say you want to launch an e-commerce business selling chocolates. Probably, you are going to design your business model around peak sales in February, since most people buy chocolates as gifts for Valentine's Day. Your sales in July and August might be minuscule, since chocolate tends to melt when it is being driven around in a hot UPS truck. On the other hand, in that landscape example, you're going to have a lot more business cutting lawns in July and August than you will in February. By seeing through your goal, you can once again anticipate the ups and downs, set goals accordingly, and have different strategies for different times.

The real skill is knowing your business just like knowing your favorite sport. If you are into football like I am, you know how much it pays to be someone like Tom Brady. He has played twenty years in the NFL, and he knows where the defense is going to be, or the precise speed of his receivers. He knows when to go fast and when to let the clock run out. The more experience you get in your business, the more you'll be able to anticipate its ebbs and flows and how to respond to them. That also means you need to understand your own skills as a player. For instance, Tom Brady is not a mobile quarterback, so his playbook isn't ever going to be filled with quarterback running plays. Instead, he makes a quick decision to pass to someone who found the open hole in the defense or calls an audible for a play that will exploit the defense's weakness. For you to find your own attainable goals, you need to know what kind of quarterback you are: take an inventory of your most valuable skills and resources and build your goals around them.

Rewarding

Don't get me wrong; our brains *love* rewards. More than that, they need those rewards as motivation to get through all the hard work. Each time our brain perceives a reward, it releases dopamine, that feel-good hormone responsible for pleasure.

Some recent studies have suggested that our brains are so wired to want that dopamine rush that they will go out of their way to encode pathways and memories that allow us to seek it out again. In other words, if we experience pleasure and accomplishment from completing a task, our brain will literally map memories and stimuli to encourage us to go down that same path again. This is why retail therapy and midnight ice cream eating habits are so hard to break and so easy to turn to in times of stress. We can actually train our brain to like things we really don't like doing because of the expected reward at the end. This rewards section must be taken seriously for two reasons: our brain needs rewards to perform at peak levels, but it can also get addicted, which will sour your motivation behind the goal. This is why I hope this chapter can help give you perspective that was, and remains, paramount when it comes to my own goals/rewards ecosystem.

In my opinion, a reward has to actually upgrade your life, rather than be something that is really just about vanity or just acquiring more stuff. Rewards should be assets in your life, not liabilities. For instance, I don't like the drudgery of just driving from point A to point B, so I set a goal for myself of having enough money to buy a high-performance sports car. I also knew that I live on a gravel road and our house doesn't have a garage, so I knew that I also needed something practical. As much fun as it would have been to have a flashy Lamborghini, that kind of car was never going to be a good idea in those conditions, and the reality of owning it was never going to be an actual upgrade in my life, since I would have been constantly paying to repair rock chips or damage done by mice chewing at very expensive wires. Instead, I bought the BMW M3: it has a higher clearance than a Lamborghini and is a lot less money to repair. It is also still a ton of fun to drive, and I arrive at work each morning filled with energy and with a giant smile on my face. What makes this car a good reward for me is that it upgrades a boring experience (in this case, commuting to work) and keeps me motivated to give my patients my all. Every time I see it and step into it, I get excited about it. Taking care of it doesn't feel like a drag, but in fact the opposite is true, because it is a true asset and helps me perform on a high level.

So how can you find the right rewards for you? Let's say you want to start a housekeeping business. Maybe you've been using your parents' basic supermarket mop and bucket, which can take a lot of time and energy to use, but you don't have the startup cash to get a fancy steam mop. You could set yourself a goal that, when you reach a certain number of clients, you're going to buy one of those fancy automated all-in-one vacuum and mop combinations that allows you to do the floors in a fraction of the time. Not only is this an upgrade because it means that you don't have to work as hard, but it will also save you time that will free you up to accept more clients. Maybe you're that stay-at-home mom with all the chores to do, but you want to start an essential oils company. You could set yourself a goal that, when you hit a certain profit, you are going to buy yourself a washing machine that can do four loads at once. That will free you up to invest more time both in your growing business project and your family members. You will remember the ease of touching one button and how great it is that the chore takes an hour, versus the days when it took all day. That will motivate you to look for other areas of your life to upgrade, and maybe even one day you'll hire a full-time housekeeper so you can just enjoy time with the kids and work on your business. Rewards can also be something as simple as a showerhead that massages achy muscles or super comfy workout gear that motivates you to hit the gym. In all of these cases, you could make do with what you have, but getting something new will make life feel that much better, and you have acquired assets that continue to help you build momentum.

Remember, we don't set goals only to get rewards. This is only sustainable if our rewards are kept, not only with the lifestyle we want to live, but also with our values and purpose. So ask yourself: how can you attach life-upgrading assets as rewards to your goals?

THE SELFISH WHY

As we talked about earlier in the book, all the great entrepreneurs are successful in part because they want to impact the world and solve problems that advance humanity. This is the selfless purpose. On the other side of the coin lies the selfish why. I know this might ruffle some feathers, but I want you to know it is okay to work and be motivated in part by what you get out of it. Even as a Christian, I sacrifice much of my earthly desires for my treasure being stored up in heaven, but I still am motivated by the primal question: "What is in it for me?" This, in my opinion, is your selfish why, and it is healthy. Sometimes this comes in the form of a reward, as we just talked about, but this is more about the feeling you get when enjoying something that your hard work made possible. It's something you aren't ashamed to share, use, talk about, or show because whatever "it" is, is merely a symbol. Maybe it's six-pack abs, a nice car, pictures of a vacation you took, your house, a garden, or literally anything that brings you meaning and brings out the warm feelings every time you experience it.

Many entrepreneurs I have talked to feel bad about talking about things they did or bought because they don't want to seem selfish or boastful. While the danger is there for that to happen, remember, the selfish why isn't the only reason why you work—it fulfills a part of the vision. You might not even need a reward for every goal achieved. My car has kept me plenty motivated, and there is little more I want right now other than to make my family happy and help fulfill their life dreams and goals. When I see my wife happy with her garden, or my daughter enjoy playing her new guitar to be like Daddy, I also consider that part of my selfish why. I enjoy the feeling I get inside when I see them happy. As we move forward, I encourage you to explore your cravings and desires and see how they might fit into helping you along as you pursue your grand vision and world-changing purpose.

CROSSING THE FINISH LINE

Once you've settled on goals within your vision that you know are personal, attainable, and rewarding, you still need a detailed plan for making that goal a reality. Here are a few best practices that have really helped me troubleshoot through tough and confusing times while building and running my business.

Work Backward (But Not Too Far Forward)

Whether it's launching a new business or saving for retirement, a long-term goal can feel intimidating, no matter how much you believe in it. To help avoid those feelings, find ways to set lots of little goals along the way. Not only will doing so provide a much-needed sense of accomplishment along the way, but it also helps you budget your time, resources, and sweat equity.

Once you've established a long-term goal (a year to five years), begin by visualizing yourself in that space. Then work backward, creating a series of identifiable subgoals all the way back to where you are now—kind of like Hansel and Gretel's trail of breadcrumbs.

No one knows how to do this better than long-distance runners. Do a quick Google search and you'll find dozens of training programs for completing your first marathon. Not a single one of them recommends that you go out and run twenty miles on your first training day. Instead, all of them work on the same basic principle: taking the known end goal of 26.2 miles, then work backward over a series of weeks, decreasing the length of your weekly long run, until you're all the way back to square one. Then, going forward, those gradual increases feel realistic and manageable, even if you've never run more than five miles at a time.

This process works for every other kind of goal as well. If your goal is to lose fifteen pounds, you may decide that, over the course of a month, you need to walk at least 600 minutes and cut at least 5,000 calories from your diet. On their face, those numbers can seem awfully overwhelming. But if you break it down by the day, we're talking about adding thirty minutes of cardio activity and cutting 200 calories. Take your dog for a bonus walk and substitute your morning white chocolate mocha with a healthier tea or just black coffee and *Bam!* You're there.

This approach works just as well in business. Say your aim is to grow your business so that it is bringing in a million dollars a year. You could break that down to first earning $500,000 or even $250,000, but those numbers can seem scary as well. Instead, keep breaking them down. How are you going to make $100,000? $10,000? Keep going until you hit a number you know you can attain. Then go forward again...

...but not too far forward. Remember, goals are there to help you achieve your dreams, not weigh you down. Thinking about the big goals can make life feel overwhelming and ultimately keep you from making forward progress. So it is important to dream big, then set small action steps to get there.

It's also important to keep your eye on the long term but your attention on the short term. The future will bring its own worries, so set a plan so you can accomplish things one step at a time. Anyone that has long-distance hiking experience can easily relate to this. I learned about it myself when I hiked Mount Whitney, the highest mountain in the lower forty-eight states. For years I had driven by the intimidating mountain on my way to other adventures, then, in 2016, a good friend was able to get the permits we needed to climb, and he invited me to come along. Driving up on the access road, I began to realize how much bigger the mountain looked from close up. We started our hike before dawn, and it was so dark we couldn't even see the trail except for what our headlamps illuminated right in front of us. As the daylight grew around us, we were halfway up the mountain and still hiking at a pretty good pace. We knew from research that the hardest part of the hike would be the last third, where the trail becomes what is known as the land of ninety-nine switchbacks, because the grade increases so dramatically that the only way up is to basically just go back and forth for what feels like a million times. At that point, the trail is just brutal: it gains about a thousand or so feet of elevation in a single mile, and the only way up is to take short little steps in order to not fully stretch your muscles, but stay within "eco mode," if you will. Even though it felt like we were shuffling, my friend and I made it to the summit before noon. When we had set out, I had no idea how or if we would make it. But by just focusing first on the tiny bit of trail illuminated by my headlamp and then, eventually, on the equally tiny stride required by the final incline, we made it—and we did so by not thinking too far forward. Personal goals can be achieved the exact same way.

Check (and Recheck) the Map

On that same Mount Whitney trip, my friend and I happened to meet a small group of rock climbers. Unlike us, they were heading straight up the mountain. Because their route was much shorter, they had left long after we did, but they still passed us. And because their route was that much shorter, they also didn't need to carry nearly as much water and food as we did. That added weight should have made us slower than the rock climbers, so my friend and I were both really surprised when, a couple of miles later, we saw the climbers once again coming up behind us. In fact, we were so surprised we asked them what had happened. Turns out, they had taken a wrong turn shortly after we first met them, and it had taken them quite a while before they realized it.

Had they stopped and looked at the map, they would have seen that they had taken the wrong fork in a path or that the lake was on their wrong side. Instead, they kept going and fell way behind and had to backtrack.

Setting and achieving your goals also requires you to keep checking your map. Doing so allows you to evaluate your progress and make any changes or fine tuning that is necessary. Say I set a goal for a number of new patients in a month. By the third weekend, I may realize we're not going to make it. At that point, either I need to create a new plan for the following month that will allow me to catch up and achieve what I couldn't this month, or I need to accept that the goal was too ambitious and re-evaluate. What I discovered during the COVID-19 pandemic is that it is sometimes just impossible to predict how achievable a goal can be: with schools yo-yoing between remote and open, my patients often had to cancel or reschedule appointments. Sports teams would practice for a while and then be canceled. I soon discovered that maybe setting a goal for total patient visits wasn't a great marker of the work that I was doing, so we decided to measure something different and not put as much emphasis on the patient volume stat. I still tracked that line on my sheet, but I chose to be conservative with it so as to not burden myself with failed metrics.

At some point in your journey, you will probably have to be equally conservative. Let's go back to our example of the landscaper. He created a scalable plan and understood the calendar variability in his profession (remember, August is *always* going to be busier for him than February). But that doesn't mean all Augusts will be created equally for him. One year, heavy rains might mean that he has to cut his clients' lawns every week or even twice a week.

Another year, drought may kill much of the grass and the majority of his clients may suspend their contracts. In both cases, his ability to adapt—either by hiring temporary workers or expanding his services—will mean the difference between a month of profit or one of loss. Remember, you set goals to help yourself not only make progress toward your dreams, but also be the canary in the coal mine. If a goal isn't being met in one area, maybe set goals for other aspects of your business that might have been overlooked.

When you make sure to evaluate your plan along the way, you are actually doing a lot of important mental work. For starters, you're taking inventory of your literal and metaphoric surroundings, which allows you to gain self-awareness and figure out where you are in the grand scheme of things. Whether we know it or not, our brains are constantly doing something similar in terms of their connection with our bodies. This process is sometimes referred to as a sixth sense; it is called *proprioception*, or the brain's ability to know where the body is in space. The brain can make this determination because all of our muscles and joints are constantly sending signals about their movements. When your body has a full range of motion, your brain has "full bars" or full reception from the body's sensors. In that case, your brain is content: it's receiving all the information it needs from the outside environment, so there's no need to frantically hunt for sensory information or to constantly warn you to do this or not to do that. Compare that to the day after a brutal squat workout. Your muscles are so sore they're screaming, and they'll do anything they can to avoid being further overtaxed. That includes sending you a pain response so that you make sure to take the elevator instead of climbing three flights of stairs.

Nociception is what your brain perceives as pain, and it will trigger a systemic stress response in an effort to survive the threat around you. If there is a lack of proper joint movement (proprioception), the brain will then be receiving nociception signals. This is why when you feel a spasm in your neck or back you want to instantly move it and stretch it. Your brain is seeking proprioception because it doesn't like nociception. I see this all the time in my patients with special needs, especially those kids with autism and ADHD. So often, I find that their vertebrae and spine aren't moving the way they should. That is part of why these patients self-mutilate or bang their heads against the wall; it's also why tight hugs or weighted blankets can soothe them—in both cases, the pressure is sending helpful sensory information to the brain, which in turn creates a much-needed awareness of what's actually going on in the kids' environment. It can also turn off their fight-or-flight stress response.

You don't have to have special needs to see this same phenomenon work in your own body. Think about what happens when your leg or arm falls asleep. If you're like me, the first thing you feel afterward is that sharp sensation of pins and needles. Why? Because your nociception is working hard to get any kind of stimulus back from your sleeping limb. Pain stimulus is better than none at all.

Every mammal has its own version of this need to know where we are in space and time. When we are having our own, human, difficulty locating ourselves in space, we may do something similar. If you've ever resorted to retail therapy to help you get through a difficult breakup or a midlife crisis, congratulations: you've proven your brain is equipped with nociception. In that case, your brain had probably grown numb from the stimulus you were sending it. By losing your sense of purpose or ability to identify and meet your goals, you basically forced part of your brain to fall asleep. That, in turn, made the rest of your brain panic because it wasn't receiving enough stimulus, so it went in search of more.

Proprioception is why we set goals—to constantly be able to feel where we are in our "vision space." If we stop hitting our goals, fail to set them, or if achieving goals isn't rewarded, we will get stagnant or stuck, and our brain will start to only get nociception or panic signals, which triggers you to start living in scarcity rather than abundance. Remember goal setting is a skill, so especially in the beginning, do make it a burden and ask for help from people who are successful at setting, achieving, and rewarding their goals.

Rely on Ranges, Not Specifics

Most businesses gauge progress with key performance indicators (known as KPIs). These are quantifiable ways of measuring growth over time. These also become increasingly important when the business has more employees than just you. However, KPIs can also feel overwhelming, and they can make you detach from your purpose and make that purpose only about achieving specific goals. I would be a bit of a hypocrite if I didn't tell you that I don't necessarily have line items of KPIs for my staff and for my performance. This is one way I am different than many other business leaders. Another is that I prefer to cast a vision, attach that vision to a purpose surrounded by core values, and then fill it with goals so that the goals themselves are enough to propel the vision and push the team along the way. When I was trying to set KPIs, I would always feel like they were micromanaging performance, and that's not what I wanted to do. It took my eyes off the big picture and put them instead on those line items.

However, with casting a vision, my purpose, goals, and selfish why are more than enough. It's also scalable because you're in a sense just multiplying what you do and adding different variables, rather than defining each and every person. It also gives employees a sense of accountability and responsibility rather than just feeling like they are drones. It allows humans to showcase their uniqueness. Don't get me wrong: there do need to be clear expectations and leadership from the vision creator. Fuzzy expectations create turmoil and tension in the office, but at Trailhead Family Chiropractic, I am able to tell my staff why I want something to happen, but I also let them figure out the best way to actually do it.

Focusing on casting a vision instead of details can also help you focus on ranges and not specifics. When it comes to hiring, that can mean that you don't have to exclude a candidate because they aren't absolutely perfect at Excel or because they don't have a specific skill. We can always train up the specific tasks (to a degree), but character and purpose are most important for me, especially being in a people business.

Unless your life's dream is to become a prizefighting welterweight, there is rarely a time when your goal needs to involve a precise figure. I fell into this trap when I set a goal of a particular number of new patients. Anything short—even just a single person—felt like a failure. If, on the other hand, I'd set myself a modest and achievable range, both me and my employees would have felt much better about the work we were doing and the effort we were putting in to get there. Maybe it's because I'm not much of a golfer, but when I was setting that goal I forgot one very important point: par for any hole can usually only happen with ideal conditions. Not even a pro is going to achieve that if he is playing in a monsoon or a blizzard.

When we fail to account for all of the normal variabilities from week to week or month to month, when we aren't experienced enough to anticipate natural ebbs and flows, we can inadvertently set ourselves up for disaster. For example, let's say your goal is to lose three pounds a month over the course of a year. That goal may work just fine for you, but once Halloween candy season rolls around, it's going to become much more difficult. By the time Thanksgiving and Christmas arrive, most people I know are happy just not to have gained three pounds, let alone losing any.

A range allows for this kind of change—and the occasional dip into your kid's plastic jack o' lantern. Those months, your goal is simply to maintain your weight, rather than to lose any additional pounds. It also means you can enjoy turkey and conversation with your family, even if it means you pass on the mashed potatoes. If, at the end of the year, you tell me you lost thirty pounds instead of your targeted thirty-six, I'm still going to tell you you did a fantastic job. Why? Because I can just about guarantee that you feel healthier, you have more energy, and your blood sugar is lower. You've dropped a couple of sizes, and I bet you feel pretty great in your new jeans. That's the thing about focusing on ranges instead of metrics: it allows our brain to focus on a mindset of abundance, and it gives us plenty of room to feel a sense of accomplishment—and often gratitude—for what we did accomplish, rather than seducing us into the failure spiral that happens when we fixate on what we didn't get done.

Another practical example of this is getting out of debt. If you are $20,000 in credit card debt, it's true that that is a specific goal (you want your balance to be zero). But where the ranges come in is how you get there. You can say that you only want to spend $50 a month eating out and use the rest of the $150 you normally spend chiseling down your debt. Why it might be good to have a range is if, one month, you want to splurge and go to a really nice restaurant with friends. If you restrict yourself to $50, you'll have to say no to your friends. If instead, you allow yourself a range, you can always make up the difference other months, or you can dedicate yourself to not getting takeout or buying cups of expensive coffee.

A mentor and very successful consultant once told me it's not always about the numbers or benchmarks; instead, it is about repeatedly doing the right thing with the right people. Growth will happen, especially if you have a big vision guiding you, and goals are helpful, but they aren't everything. The takeaway from this chapter is just to plan and execute the next logical step, and what we will talk about next is how to celebrate the wins in a congruent and practical way.

Cultivate Adaptability

COVID-19 has forced us all to make changes great and small, from social distancing and grocery deliveries, to remote learning and often very painful decisions to furlough employees or close businesses altogether. For many people, weathering the pandemic has been an exercise in adapting to the new normal and finding ways to thrive within that environment.

Few of us could have planned for a crisis of the scale of COVID-19. But those individuals and businesses that were able to remain fluid and find ways to pivot during lockdowns and ongoing social-distancing mandates found a new kind of resiliency that allowed them to continue to meet their goals and operate within their lived value system.

In my personal practice, I meet many of my new patients by providing free health workshops in my community. When all activities stopped in California, so did that marketing strategy. Instead of just relying on government money and hoping things would get back to normal soon, I invented new ways to spread the word about my work. I gave my workshops as webinars and started using influencer marketing strategies that actually helped me grow 30 percent. Many companies, like mine, used this crisis as an opportunity to grow and invent new offerings for their businesses. Uber shifted many of its ride-share drivers to its UberEats platform. The national restaurant chain Chipotle hired on digital-only kitchens in response to the pandemic and saw a big increase in profits as a result. On a more local level, a friend of mine owns a party rental business that specializes in events like birthday parties and weddings. With no market for bouncy houses and chocolate fountains, he began looking for other revenue streams. He quickly discovered the restaurants, churches, and gyms were all searching for outdoor tents that would allow them to maintain distancing protocols. He grew his tent inventory and offered specials on installations and long-term rentals.

In no time, he had work for all of his employees and monthly earnings that rivaled those of his pre-pandemic business.

Stories like this are all around the country right now: restaurants that applied for and received grants to make boxed lunches for healthcare workers; concert venues and movie theaters offering drive-up experiences; pop-up shops in parking garages. We can all learn a lot from these tales of success. Goals are great, but we must be ready to revise or even abandon and replace them when the situation calls.

Keep this in mind with your own goals, no matter how small or large.

CHAPTER 5

THE ESSENTIALS

A FEW YEARS AGO, MY MOM AND I WENT BACKPACKING TOGETHER.
If you've ever been on a similar adventure, you know that a reliable, lightweight stove is an essential piece of gear. I have a little
one that I always bring with me, and one of the things I love the
most is that it has a convenient internal starter that lights a little
spark to ignite the fuel. Rule number one before going out into
the wilderness is to test your gear, check for holes, and things
like that, but neither of us really took a look at all of it before we
set out, and we'd made it up above 10,000 feet before we took a
break and were ready to cook our meal. I set up my trusty stove,
but when I went to click on the self-lighting apparatus, nothing
happened. I tried again: still nothing. I was beginning to think we
were going to have to eat granola bars for dinner and didn't know
what we were going to do for the next couple of nights (I was also
mourning over the potential loss of my coffee) because I had no
other way to light the stove. Now, my mom had borrowed her

sister's backpacking kit, and she desperately looked through it for some source of a spark. In her pack, my mom found a little plastic box filled with the basic survival essentials, including matches and a lighter. Thank goodness! Because of the preparedness of my aunt, we were able to eat our hot meal and continue our trip. I learned a lesson that day to always be prepared and have multiple ways to solve a problem just in case your main way fails. This chapter is that little plastic box filled with key tools needed to solve the problems you will encounter along the way to setting and achieving your goals.

WHY THE PROBLEM ISN'T THE PROBLEM

Oftentimes in my practice a patient will come in with lower back pain caused by what they thought was a weightlifting injury or turning funny. Most doctors would treat only the area of pain, not ever knowing if the pain was in the place of the actual problem or if the root cause in another area was causing the low back pain. As I mentioned before, the testing that we do in my office gives us unique insight into the nervous system to actually identify the source of stress. I would say at least half of the time, the source of the patient's low back pain actually started in their neck, which is often why other treatment methods didn't solve the issue. This idea is the basis of this chapter: oftentimes what we think is the problem is actually only a symptom, and we need to dig into other areas of the situation to actually uncover and solve the problem at the root cause. Let me give you some examples:

- You pledged to leave your office job in six months and pursue your dream of opening a microbrewery, but a year later you haven't made it any further than sharing a few home-brewed bottles of IPA with your friends.

- You swore this was going to be the year you stopped smoking, and maybe you even made it through the whole month of January without a cigarette. But stress at work or at home had you lighting up again by spring.

- Maybe you finally invested into that network marketing business but months later still haven't sold one unit, let alone paid for the startup costs.

I get it. Even when we feel confident in our new direction and vision and feel energized by this new purpose, actualizing a goal is hard. There are so many reasons why we don't succeed. When we feel like we are failing, most people respond in one of two ways: either they throw in the towel and give up entirely, or they decide they must start over and completely reinvent the wheel. I'm here to tell you there is a much better way. But first, let's make sure there's not a different perspective you just haven't yet considered. Here's a quick scan you can practice at home by simply asking yourself a few quick questions:

- Are you just frustrated because achieving your goal is taking longer than you thought? Check in with your purpose.

- Has that purpose changed at all? If so, your goals may need to change as well.

- Evaluate your plan. Are there any incongruities preventing you from achieving your goal?

Another great idea when you hit a rough patch is to test whether you are simply facing a little adversity or a sign that this isn't the path for you. What I do is ask: Is my mind still energized by the vision? Does the end goal and vision give me goosebumps and bring a smile to my face? If you answer no to these sorts of question, despite your efforts to vet your idea, you may have started this venture without a strong enough purpose, thus giving you weak motivation, meaning you should reevaluate or take a break.

My wife Jess and I just had an experience with this while materializing my career outside of chiropractic. I thought of myself as a business consultant, helping people to get to the root cause of their business issues. When I began writing this book, I assumed I would be writing it mainly for aspiring entrepreneurs and stuck CEOs. I knew I could provide a lot of value to them, but what never quite felt right about that plan was that I knew some clients or readers would come expecting that I would make their business's bottom line better through sales and marketing techniques. I probably could help with that, but only as a byproduct of the real work I would want to do with them, which is helping them to become better people. I explained this problem to Jess the other night and she said, "So you mean you're more of a mentor?" And that's when it really hit me: business consultants spend a lot of their time working with marketing plans and advertising; what I want to do is help people live in their purpose. So the problem wasn't actually about me figuring out a way to do that work as a business consultant; it was that I had to shift the branding and business model to more of a mentorship relationship. As I thought about how I would monetize that, I was constantly hitting the wall. Then, on a random evening, listening to a book while driving, it came to me: I am a six-figure small business strategist for service-based professionals who want to regain freedom while making more money, just as I have. Now everything makes sense, and every time I want to give up, I ask myself those questions and know that I have to keep pushing through the struggle until I figure it out.

If you find yourself butting your head against the wall over and over and over again, instead of trying to figure out a way to go through it, look around and you might discover that there is a door. Just that little change in perspective can prevent you from getting a nasty headache and can save you lots of time and money. Oftentimes, if you just look left or right, you're going to most likely find a much easier way to go instead of just being so focused on *this is the way.*

As a species, we all suffer from some version of what scholar and author Dan Heath refers to as *problem blindness.* In his book *Upstream,* Heath describes a company that seemed to have everything going for it: great customer satisfaction, an outstanding workplace environment, and a genuinely happy and productive staff. But because every team within their company was focused on its own objectives and outcomes (sales, customer service, technology, etc.), no one noticed that their online business was spending millions of dollars a year on customer support. The whole point of having an online business is to *reduce* staff needs, so why was there such demand for customer support if the reviews were constantly positive? Turns out, most customers were calling to see if their order was received, so they started sending out automated emails which confirmed their order. The result? Millions of dollars in savings on reduced customer service needs.

As Heath describes, there wasn't necessarily anything wrong with the way things were going, as customers were happy, but that small tweak in the system made everybody happier. Oftentimes we do the same in our business or even relationships. We try to tinker with the symptoms instead of addressing the root cause behind the symptoms.

Another problem entrepreneurs face is pride. We become fixated on an idea or belief, even when all evidence suggests it is the wrong one. We also love easy answers, especially when they confirm what we think we already know. As a result, a lot of us walk around with what psychologists call *confirmation bias:* we look for excuses to believe what we want, even when it has us trying to jam square pegs into round holes. I see this all the time in my practice.

A new patient arrives with an extra-large Starbucks coffee, complaining about untreatable heartburn, or they want a quick adjustment to fix ten years of chronic pain. In both cases, they're totally missing the actual cause of their discomfort, which means we're both going to be hard-pressed to alleviate it.

The truth of the matter is that so much of our culture is set up around treating symptoms, rather than addressing the true problem. Most medical doctors are trained to view problems from a *pathogenic* perspective. In other words, their education as medical doctors focused on studying disease and minimizing its impacts. If a patient arrives complaining about knee pain, for instance, a pathogenic approach might be to prescribe an anti-inflammatory or to inject the patient with steroids. This might minimize the pain, but it won't address the root cause.

Chiropractic care, on the other hand, focuses on a *salutogenic* approach, a holistic approach that looks to create optimal health, rather than focusing on minimizing disease. A *salutogenic* approach to that patient with knee pain will begin by examining what is causing the inflammation and disease. Is the patient, for instance, consuming a diet high in refined sugars like corn syrup, trans fats, or alcohol? All of these have been found to increase inflammation in the body while also preventing the body from actualizing natural anti-inflammatories like omega-3 fats. We might then conduct a gait analysis and evaluate the patient's posture. Could it be that the person has flat feet that cause her to overpronate? If so, the mere fact that her feet roll in is causing her entire body to fall out of alignment. Something as simple as orthotics in her shoes can solve the problem. It could be that she suffers from particularly tight hamstring muscles, and that a combination of stretching and adjustments will help her properly realign her body or some strengthening exercises will allow her muscles to better support her knee joints.

This salutogenic approach can help you determine why you're failing to meet your goals, reveal problem blindness, and fix problems at the root cause. So next time you find yourself dealing with a problem over and over again, it might be time to stop and think holistically about your business, relationship, health, or whatever other situation you are in, and think, maybe this problem isn't *the problem*.

BRICK BY BRICK

Goals happen best when we take them one step at a time and work to establish good systems along the way. This tool is a hard one to use for me, personally. Just the other day, I was guilty of trying to accomplish forty different things at once instead of just taking it one step at a time.

One of the most popular workshops I offer is on the gut-brain connection. There, I talk about the problem with modern foods and the missing link behind almost every health issue. I talk about gluten and refined sugar and genetically modified organisms and grass-fed livestock and everything in between. But arguably the most important thing I tell my audience is this: *do not go home and change everything about your lifestyle.* That alone can place your body in a significant state of stress. Instead, try removing just gluten and dairy and keeping everything else constant. If that doesn't work, cut out caffeine and alcohol as well. Then maybe it's time to try acupuncture or a controlled fast.

The same thing happens when people come to my office with debilitating back pain. They are in so much discomfort that they are willing to try anything and to try it all at once. The fact is, it's possible to do too much to your body if you try it all at once, even if each thing you are trying is beneficial on its face. Add or remove with control, so that you can assess the results and avoid placing your body in a state of stress simply because of all the change you're throwing at it.

Similarly, changes that impact your psychological, emotional, and financial health are also best met with a staged approach. For instance, maybe you have been married for ten years and all of the little annoyances have been adding up. Some couples might just decide that their marriage is ruined and they should just walk away right now. Others might decide that they could unpack those annoyances brick by brick and save their marriage. Let's say you are up to your gills with frustration for your wife, and it seems like there is just one problem after another. It might be time to have a candid conversation and ask, "What is one thing I can start doing differently?" You can't change everything all at once, and it's not fair to expect that someone can. But maybe your wife will say she wishes you would hang up your towel every morning. And you can tell her that you want her to put the toilet paper on the opposite way. As dumb as that may sound, by doing those little things over and over again, it reinforces that you care about your spouse and want to make things work. After a month of doing that one little thing, you will gain momentum and can tackle something else.

It could be the same thing with your other family members. If you have a poor relationship with your father or your son, try beginning by setting aside some time to do something you both love. Maybe you just go to a baseball game and just sit there: you don't have to say anything to one another; you can just enjoy being in each other's company. Then, next time, you can go to a movie and afterward have a conversation strictly about what you liked about the movie. You don't always have to go for the jugular and address the really big issues. Instead, get used to liking being around somebody and doing things with somebody first. It's so easy to focus on what's wrong with somebody, and then we lose track of what we actually liked about them in the first place.

Taking one step at a time to acknowledge you care and your love for somebody else reinforces that the relationship is not just going down a black hole. Once you gain momentum and you get the hang of it and things start to go better, it's best to establish systems so that it's not all dependent on you and you can continue to other things. For example, when I wanted to set up my practice, I knew I wasn't going to be a receptionist full time, but I still had to know how to do it so I could train somebody how to do it. When we first started, I was still answering the phone about a third of the time. I had to overhear conversations so that I could make sure I could answer questions and that the new receptionists weren't saying things wrong. Once we knew the right answers and responses, we could develop a script: that way, I could be completely away from the front desk and whatever I would say would be written in a document and all the receptionist would have to do is look at that document. That section of my business could then be decentralized and not dependent on what I would say. Every once in a while, my receptionists still get questions they can't answer, but for the most part, that part of Trailhead runs on autopilot. The more you can do something similar in your business and, really, in other parts of your life, the better. Let's say that every person who reads this book wants to call me and ask a question. As much as I wish I could answer all of them, there's no way that's going to be sustainable for me. That's why my goal is to walk you through this process one step at a time and then teach you how to do what I do and how to think like I think, so then you can go do it on your own. That's the power of establishing systems: you're not tangled up with ropes that are tied to a million different projects and people; instead, you enable other people to grow.

I think the best example of this is with kids. There are reasons why sometimes you want to let your kid fall off the chair that you've told them not to stand on a million times. Because once they fall, they're probably not going to die. The worst that will happen is maybe they have to get stitches, which isn't fun, and obviously I'm not promoting children getting hurt. But if they fall down and get stitches, they are going to decide for themselves not to stand on that chair anymore because they now know the consequences. This means you can go do dishes or be outside away from the kids because you trust their decision-making skills a little bit more. It's the same thing with sports. Coaches don't tell football players every single little step they should do, and they are not continuously telling every single player where to be or whether or not to tackle the ball carrier. Instead, they teach the players to recognize and respond to certain formations. That was one reason I watched so much film in high school: so that, when the opposing team lined up a certain way, I knew how to expect a certain play and what the other players were going to do. I didn't have to react blindly to a cut right or left. That's the power of systems.

The more systems you have, the more benefits of freedom you have. And then that also empowers others to grow and be stronger and to do things that they otherwise wouldn't do if you were just going to continually solve the problems for them. Plus, the more little successes we have, the more motivated we are to have even more success and the more we begin to build a bigger picture. I call this the rainbow effect: If you see a red arch, it's just a red arch. But if you then add orange and yellow and other colors, you'll begin to see that the colors complement each other and form something far more impressive. A red arch in the sky is pretty cool, but a rainbow is a big marvel. If you can find beauty in the little things that you do, recognize that putting them all together is going to actually make something magnificent. In other words, layered success equals ultimate success.

CLEAN OUT THE CLUTTER

Minimalist TV shows have taken the world by storm. From tiny homes to bringing joy into your home and removing everything else, clearing out the clutter in life has taken center stage, and for good reason: clutter adds complexity. To understand how it works, think about the last time you attempted to assemble a 500-piece jigsaw puzzle. Probably, you started by dumping all of the pieces onto the table and then turning them right-side up. If you're like me, next you probably lined up all of the corner and edge pieces. After that, you probably grouped pieces by color. Problem solving works this way, too.

The reason so many of us start with the edge pieces is that they are clearly identifiable by one or two flat sides, so we immediately have a good guess of where they might go. Once those edge pieces are all connected, we have a tidy border that lets us make other connections, all of which are much easier than just trying to connect random pieces, hoping they are a match. Those corner and edge pieces create a boundary and also help us to group the remaining pieces. We can tell by looking that the top right may have red in it and the top left has more yellow. So we can begin to focus our energies on figuring out in what general area the remaining pieces might go. Once you figure out where all of the red pieces go, you can move on to the yellow pieces, all the while knowing where your attention is going to go and how to work most efficiently

Your purpose and your values are a whole lot like the completed puzzle. The corners and edges of that puzzle are the goals that give your purpose shape and form. Once those are in place, you can be intentional about figuring where everything else goes—as well as what doesn't belong. It's about prioritizing your time and consolidating your tasks so that you can figure out what to focus on and when.

Let me give you an example of this from my own life. In high school, I was the pole vaulter for our track and field team. It takes a lot of mental focus to run as fast as you can, jam a long stick into a tiny hole, and let yourself be catapulted through space as you hope and pray that you fall on the intended padded mat. To get to the place where I could do this again and again without having a nervous breakdown, I developed a mental exercise to help me concentrate. Basically, I'd picture a room with layers and layers of awful old wallpaper—the busy 1960s kind with all the crazy geometric shapes and patterns. Before each competition, I'd close my eyes and imagine myself peeling off that paper layer by layer until all that was left were clean white walls. By the time I was done, my mind felt settled and relaxed, a blank slate that could concentrate entirely on my next vault.

For some people, this clearing of the clutter can be an entirely mental exercise. For others, it involves creating a work or living space conducive to fostering focus and prioritization. For some people, that means letting dishes pile up in the sink for a day or two so that they can focus on a project. For others, it might mean knocking out the dishes first so that they're not distracted by wondering when they'll get done. The important thing is that you know how many puzzle pieces you have and a rough idea of where they might go.

Here's another example from my own life. The other day, I had to get my car smogged. I hate having to do this: the places are small and dirty, and they have zero customer service because getting your car smogged is a mandated rule in California. You have to go get it done no matter what, so there is no motivation for them to provide a good experience. On the day I planned to bring in my BMW, I made sure to call one of the inspection stations to see how long their wait time was. The guy said there was no wait time, so I told him I'd be there in fifteen minutes. When I got there, I walked in the door and couldn't even figure out where the front desk was or if I was even in the right place. I finally found one of the employees and told him I was the guy who had called fifteen minutes earlier. He responded by telling me that there was going to be an hour wait. I tried to explain that I'd just called and they'd told me there wasn't any wait, but it didn't seem to matter. I told him I would leave and come back later, but he said if I didn't just leave the car, it was probably going to take even longer. By then, I was so frustrated I just left and decided to find another inspection station.

As I was driving away, I began to wonder why there wasn't just a mobile smog service that could come to you, like so many windshield replacement companies do. That got me thinking: what would it take to create a mobile service that could drive to wherever people worked and test their cars' emissions there? I began to lay out all the different factors. You'd need all of the testing equipment, along with a trailer to get it to different locations. You probably need training and some kind of certification to perform the tests. Before I knew it, I had begun to create a business plan for this niche industry that I knew nothing about. But I was able to figure it out because I knew the basic borders and corner pieces for a successful business, and I also knew how to focus in and organize the remaining details.

Clutter can manifest itself in emotional forms as well. If your marriage is in trouble or you're in a particularly rough patch with a child or parent or friend, that psychological energy is going to clutter up every other aspect of your life until you either patch up the relationship or find another form of closure.

If you're an empath like me, it's hard not to absorb all the energy of people around you. After a particularly taxing day of helping patients in need, I can definitely feel weighed down by their collective suffering. I've had to create my own rituals to make sure I don't bring that home to my relationships with my family. Some of these rituals include creating a clearly defined space where I meet with my patients. After any appointment, I walk through a series of literal dividers back to my office. Thinking of them as energy dividers—places where I leave my patients' pain or discomfort—has really helped me resist the urge to carry around their collective discomfort.

You can find your own visualizations that help you shrug off energy that belongs to other people. Ultimately, it doesn't matter whether you're bringing the stress of home to work or the stress of work to home. Either way, you may as well be toting an industrial-sized bag of garbage with the intention of dumping it all over the place. No one wants that. So do your emotional housekeeping first, then move on to your other goals.

GET OUTSIDE YOUR BOX

You've probably heard the term *devil's advocate* before but haven't thought much about its origin. The phrase actually comes from an early sixteenth-century religious tradition: whenever a person was nominated for sainthood in the Catholic Church, one high-ranking priest was appointed to argue against the person's candidacy. The idea wasn't to bring down a deserving individual but, instead, to make sure the clergy had done their job by considering every possible side of the argument. Playing devil's advocate is a great way to check yourself for both problem bias and confirmation bias.

Sometimes, playing devil's advocate can be as simple as considering the experience from your customer's perspective. When I was in school, one of my part-time jobs was working at a smoothie store. I took to heart the idea that we shouldn't make customers wait, so I'd whip up an order in pit crew time and slam down finished smoothies as fast as I could. Technically, there was nothing wrong with what I was making: the smoothies had the right ingredients, they were the right size, and they came with a lid and a straw. But in my rush to get customers their orders, I totally lost sight of the fact that I was often pouring as much smoothie down the side of the cups as I was inside of it. Customers were greeted with a dripping, sticky cup and would usually resort to grabbing a handful of napkins to wipe off their orders before picking them up. That, of course, took time. So we still had customer pileups, not to mention very sticky counters, used napkins all over the place, and empty napkin dispensers that constantly had to be refilled. What I thought was efficiency actually created a huge mess.

Even the best-intentioned ideas will fail miserably if they aren't considered from the customers' perspective. You may remember Frito Lay's decision to make their SunChips bags 100 percent compostable. It was a great idea on paper, but the bag was so loud that customers stopped purchasing them, even though the bag was a real innovation in sustainable packaging.

On the other hand, some ideas may seem frivolous on paper but more than pay for themselves when it comes to customer satisfaction and return business. After recently experiencing a problem with the new wheels on my car, I scheduled an appointment at a BMW dealership. I could have gone to one of those aftermarket places and gotten them done cheaper, but I decided to go to the dealership because I knew they were famous for really quality customer service. The place was immaculate, and the service manager greeted me by name when I arrived. Inside, it wasn't some dirty waiting room with a bunch of Goodwill chairs like a lot of mechanics have. Instead, they had leather chairs and the floors were mopped; they had fresh coffee and complimentary bananas.

As part of their service package, the dealership offers a complimentary twenty-two-point safety inspection. They complete it with a video that shows customers parts of their cars that they have probably never seen, including the undercarriage and their actual fluid levels. As the mechanic completes the inspection, he walks around with the camera and tells customers exactly what they are looking at. Do some customers toss out those images without ever looking at them? Maybe. But even just receiving them can instill confidence. For me, having a narrated video included me in the experience and helped me get to know my car better. It also made me trust the mechanic and the dealership more because I was learning about their process and the way my car works. They also booked and paid for an Uber for me so that I could get back to work. All of these little touches showed that they really cared about customer experience and want to be at the top of their game. By the time I got to work the day of that appointment, I was literally thinking about how we could do the same at Trailhead.

Another way to think about this idea of being a devil's advocate is *thinking outside the box*. Let me give you an example from my practice. A while ago, we were struggling to find ways to accommodate new clients. We wanted to make each appointment worthwhile and to ensure that all of our patients were getting the personalized attention that distinguishes the Trailhead practice. But despite our best efforts, we kept encountering inefficiencies in the use of examination and treatment space that prevented us from increasing the number of patients we saw in any one day. Meanwhile, patients were experiencing inconvenient wait times, both in our reception area and at our adjustment tables. I contacted my mentors and other leaders in the chiropractic world, looking for solutions. They admitted they were all stuck on the same issues as well. I started to think that perhaps Trailhead had just reached its patient cap.

I didn't come up with a solution to this problem until I got my hair cut. It wasn't the actual shortening of my hair length that helped me solve the problem; it's what I observed happening inside the shop. I was amazed at the productivity happening around me. I asked the stylist cutting my hair about it, and she explained their model: multiple chairs that allowed the stylists to move from station to station during what would otherwise be downtime. For example, after applying color to one client's hair, a stylist could then go shampoo another person. While someone was sitting under the drying hood, their stylist could be giving a cut to someone like me. Just buying those extra chairs and using one client's processing time as an opportunity to provide another service had radically increased the salon's productivity. I saw in an instant how this same strategy could be applied to Trailhead's business model as well. Did I expect the solution to come from a hair salon? Of course not. But I am always thinking about my business and how to make it better, so I knew I could take this system and make it work for my chiropractic practice as well. Cross-cultural collaboration can provide all kinds of pathways into new solutions as well as different angles you otherwise might never have thought about.

Having been to hundreds of chiropractic seminars and lectures, you would think I learned how to run a good business. In some ways I did, but it wasn't until I started attending lectures and reading books from entrepreneurs in other fields that I really considered myself a CEO of a business. I know this is the same for many service professionals: whether it's plumbers, electricians, personal trainers, etc., most individuals tend to try and learn only from the best in their field. The most elite, successful chiropractors run two-million-dollar clinics, give or take. If I only learned from my profession, I would probably learn how to run up to a two-million-dollar clinic or group of clinics. While that is a great income, there are entrepreneurs making many more millions than that! While it is great to learn from your friends and colleagues, I recommend you also learn from someone making more money on a bigger scale, whether they are in your profession or not. It will help you make more money, and save you money on the ignorance tax.

Don't be afraid of opposing opinions; in fact, it can be super helpful to ask the opinion of someone who you know disagrees with you. If you are starting your essential oils business and are new to oils, it would be a good idea to ask that person who thinks they are worthless their thoughts. This person will ask you questions your friends won't and give you a perspective your team can't. Don't take criticism personally, especially if it aligns with a greater purpose. Some people just can't see what you see, and it isn't worth arguing. It is, however, helpful to word and craft your marketing strategies to curb those objections from potential customers.

VISUALIZE SUCCESS

When I talk about visualization, I'm not referring to it in some kind of new-age, name it and claim type of context. Instead, I'm talking about actually charting out what meeting your goal will look like, how you're going to get there, and what kind of terrain you're going to encounter along the way.

That last element is important: walking five miles on a gravel road in Iowa is much easier than covering that same distance in the Himalayas. If you don't know what kind of elevation gains you're dealing with or what obstacles may be in your way, you'll have no idea how strenuous your journey is going to be—or even how to pack and dress for the conditions. That's one reason I love topographical maps so much: they don't just tell me where I'm going; they also tell me the easiest route to get there. Sometimes, that means going around a big hill instead of over it. Doing so may add mileage, but it'll also be quicker in the long run, and a whole lot less strenuous.

Recently, Jess and I attended a weekend homesteader conference in Tennessee. We booked an Airbnb for the family and invited her parents to join us. The four of us flew into Nashville and caught an Uber that took us pretty much straight to the place where we were going to be staying. Jess's parents, on the other hand, drove their RV from out west. Once we got settled, we called them and asked how long they would be. They said they only had two hours to go, which wasn't that bad, so we decided to get dinner and wait up for them. After about three and a half hours had gone by, Jess's parents still hadn't arrived. We called them again to find out where they were, and they told us that their GPS said they still had an hour to go. We couldn't believe it. We asked them if they were caught in traffic or if there had been an accident, but they said no, they just kept having to take a bunch of turns. The GPS didn't know they were in a giant motorhome, and it kept sending them on these side roads with sharp hairpin turns and not a lot of visibility, which meant they kept having to back up, turn a little, back up, turn a little, and on and on. That also meant they were going much, much slower than what the GPS predicted. The same thing happened to us later in the conference: we plugged a route into the GPS, and it took us out into all of this wide-open property. The GPS kept telling us we only had five minutes left in our drive, but fifteen minutes later, we were still driving around and making all of these turns to the left and to the right. Jess and I were both like, *what the heck?* We could see our destination on the map, but the GPS was sending us on the most round-about way that was technically less mileage but way longer than if we had gone the straight route. We didn't really understand that before we arrived in Tennessee, since California has so many freeways and is always going to be faster because of how many traffic lights and stop signs are on city streets. If we had looked ahead at our route, we might have realized that what our GPS said was the quickest route wasn't really.

Life can work the same way if we aren't careful to draw out our vision and goals. Personally, I use a flow chart every time I come up with a new idea so I can see the whole process from a bird's-eye view. Most of the time I realize there are pitfalls and gaps I need to fill in before moving forward that I probably would have missed if I just rushed into things. A flow chart also invites other people into your thought process, kind of like common core math, so they can see your work and where you want to go. Remember that story of the janitor that solved the impossible math question on the chalkboard? Someone can do that to your problem too if you just get it out of your head and show your work. Let me teach you how the process of working through a flow chart works.

Place a sheet of paper in front of you in the landscape orientation. On the far right-hand side of the page, write your goal. On the far left side is your starting point. In between, chart the steps you are going to take to get from one side to the other.

Flowchart: What Is It?

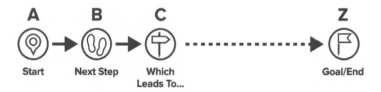

A	B	C		Z
Start	Next Step	Which Leads To...		Goal/End

Say your goal is to get out of bad debt. The benefits extend far beyond just an improved credit score. They also include the emotional relief of ending the stress of knowing your life is owned by someone else and the shame that can come from not being able to get a car loan or mortgage for a new house. To accomplish this, consider setting yourself a goal that, no matter how hard to achieve, will come with equal amounts of happiness, like paying cash for a family vacation to Hawaii. Now, what are the steps you're going to need to get there? Most likely they are going to revolve around decreasing your spending and increasing your income. So maybe your flow chart has two parallel tracks, one for each step. The spending thread could include tasks like unsubscribing from apps that include a fee (those monthly charges for $2.99 add up a lot faster than you might think), along with streaming service add-ons like premium channels. The chart for your income may include taking on a part-time job or finding ways to monetize tasks you already enjoy doing, like snowplowing or tutoring on the side.

Example: Out of Debt

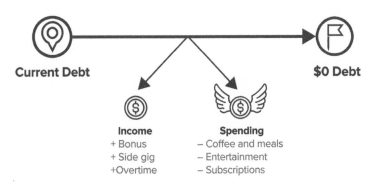

Current Debt $0 Debt

Income
+ Bonus
+ Side gig
+Overtime

Spending
– Coffee and meals
– Entertainment
– Subscriptions

I have also written out a personal example I used to streamline
and improve my practice experience:

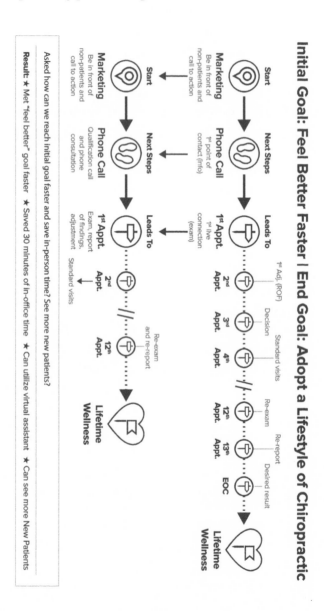

Initial Goal: Feel Better Faster | End Goal: Adopt a Lifestyle of Chiropractic

Start → **Next Steps** → **Leads To**

Marketing
Be in front of
non-patients and
call to action

Phone Call
1st point of
contact (info)

1st Appt.
1st live
connection
(exam)

Start → **Next Steps** → **Leads To**

Marketing
Be in front of
non-patients and
call to action

Phone Call
Qualification call
and phone
consultation

1st Appt.
Exam, report
of findings,
adjustment

1st Adj. (ROF) → Decision → Standard visits → Re-exam → Re-report

2nd Appt. / 3rd Appt. / 4th Appt. / 12th Appt. / 13th Appt. / EOC — Desired result — **Lifetime Wellness**

Standard visits

2nd Appt. — Re-exam and re-report — 12th Appt.

Lifetime Wellness

Asked how can we reach initial goal faster and save in-person time? See more new patients?

Result: ★ Met "feel better" goal faster ★ Saved 30 minutes of in-office time ★ Can utilize virtual assistant ★ Can see more New Patients

Finally, here is an example of how you can map out a weight loss journey:

Example: Lose Weight

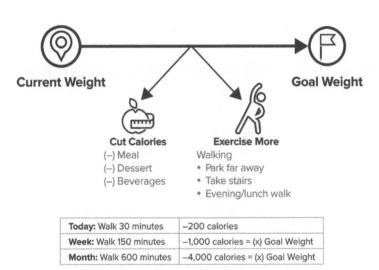

Current Weight **Goal Weight**

Cut Calories
(–) Meal
(–) Dessert
(–) Beverages

Exercise More
Walking
• Park far away
• Take stairs
• Evening/lunch walk

Today: Walk 30 minutes	–200 calories
Week: Walk 150 minutes	–1,000 calories = (x) Goal Weight
Month: Walk 600 minutes	–4,000 calories = (x) Goal Weight

Mapping out each step lets you understand the topography before you, and just how much effort traversing it will require. It'll demonstrate where the truly strenuous parts of your journey lie and good places to either set up a base camp or bivouac for the night. If that metaphor doesn't resonate with you, think of the flow chart as a series of railroad cars strung together, with each boxcar representing a step in your progress. The beautiful thing about this exercise is that you have nearly limitless choices for how you're going to set up your train. An engine can haul one giant car filled with coal, but it's going to be more efficient if you divide that coal amongst several cars. The chart also works wonders for figuring out how you are spending your time and where efficiencies can best be discovered.

Personally, I'm a whiteboard guy. When I'm stumped or in a jam, I'll grab a handful of dry erase markers and sketch out ideas and solutions until I finally find the way out. It can be a sloppy process with a lot of arrows and scribbles but, in the end, I'm always excited to see a solution looking back at me. If you're using paper, be sure to use a pencil with a giant eraser. Start over whenever you don't like the look of your chart, and don't be afraid to try a new course. The great thing about this process is that absolutely nothing is permanent. And the more you practice this technique, the sooner working solutions will manifest themselves.

The same is true for the other tools in this chapter. The more you practice them, the more adept you'll become at using each of them. Just as importantly, you'll become that much more skilled at knowing which tool any situation requires. For instance, over time it will become almost instinctively apparent to you whether a situation is best solved by playing devil's advocate or clearing out the clutter. Ultimately, though, when it comes to trouble-shooting when you aren't meeting your personal goal, it doesn't matter what tool you grab, so long as it is one that gets you closer to where you're trying to go.

PRACTICE MAKES PERMANENT

Hopefully those essentials have you prepared to tackle your problems when you encounter them and you at least have the ability to ask yourself better questions. Oftentimes at semi-nars or with coaches, I never really knew what questions to ask because I honestly didn't know what my problem was. These strategies are the few I have developed to help me solve the prob-lem myself, or go to a mentor with an actionable question. This is how you can actually get into conversation with some of these master problem solvers: Ask actionable questions. Show them on paper, walk them through your failures and what you have already tried. Most importantly, always remember your purpose so you don't get stuck in the details. Oftentimes the details mean much less to your customers and those around you than they do to you. Don't get me wrong, I appreciate the details, and if you ever come visit my practice, or use me as your strategist, you will experience it for yourself, but I don't let the details stop me from moving forward. Everyone will care less about your business than you, so don't take it personally. Remember your purpose; practice asking better questions; and take time to brainstorm, plan, and execute separately to avoid feeling overwhelmed. Finally, be vulnerable with others, especially if these strategies are new to you. Don't throw pearls before swine, but also take into consideration when multiple people think your idea isn't right just yet, especially if those people carry heavy emotional weight in your life. Nothing we do will ever be perfect, but how we do everything eventually can become permanent, so practice problem solving in a way that is sustainable and healthy for the future and the present.

CHAPTER 6

PERSPECTIVE

I BEGAN THIS BOOK WITH MY OWN ROCK BOTTOM STORY: HOW I had forgotten my purpose and dismissed my values in pursuit of quick professional and financial growth. As I mentioned in those introductory pages, the real problem I suffered from was a lack of congruence. In this last chapter, let's explore more about what a congruent life looks like and why it is so important for achieving your goals.

Most likely, you first encountered the word *congruence* in a high school geometry class, when you were probably asked to identify the two triangles that were mirror images of each other. The idea of a congruent lifestyle comes from the same idea. The word *congruent* comes from the Latin word for "agreement" or "harmony." A congruent life is one in which all of your daily choices, both large and small, are in keeping with your purpose and values.

Making a choice that is incongruent with our values knocks us out of alignment and will eventually lead to you living in a continual state of stress. Sometimes, making these decisions causes us to sacrifice some experiences, but for the greater good of our purpose. One example in my life is that I made the personal choice not to drink alcohol in college. I knew that a single DUI would cost me my license, ending my career as a chiropractor and taking me away from my selfless purpose.

Living a congruent lifestyle means maintaining a disciplined mindset in keeping with your values and purpose. This can be an easy idea to forget, especially when the demands of everyday life start to build up around us, or we experience peer pressure from friends or relatives, or "short-cuts to success" scams come our way. It's easy to succumb to resentment, anger, envy, or even an inflated sense of our own worth. When diagnosing those feelings, you can usually pin them on the difference between your reality and your expectations of reality. As much as I'd love to say I'm immune to those moments, it's simply not true. The summer before I left for the University of Montana, I took a job working at an ice cream parlor chain. I had already committed to becoming a chiropractor and had trained my mind to think about living the lifestyle of a doctor. Ice cream parlors are notoriously messy, sticky places, and this one was no different. Cleaning our ice cream maker was a disgusting chore, and I can vividly remember one night when it was my turn to clean it. The drain behind the machine had overflowed, and I was on my hands and knees, covered in melted ice cream and the grime that accumulates in a busy restaurant. It was late, I was exhausted from a long shift, and all I could think was, *this job is totally beneath me.* I was certain I was destined for a far more prestigious career and all the perks that come along with it. I couldn't wait to be a doctor and leave these lowly chores behind me, I thought.

I'd almost forgotten about that moment entirely when I finally graduated from chiropractic school and began practicing. My first office was a suite in a commercial building that shared a restroom with neighboring businesses. We took turns cleaning the space, and one day it was my job to clean the restroom right after someone had had a major blowout. There I was, a newly minted doctor, cleaning one of the most disgusting toilets I'd ever encountered. While I did, I had a vivid flashback to that night cleaning the ice cream maker. I'd sworn I'd never be in such a menial position again, and there I was in one that was far worse.

That's when it hit me: I'd been so focused that I'd forgotten that the very heart of chiropractic work is to be of service. My purpose as a chiropractor is to serve my patients so that they can enjoy good health and a better life. My purpose as a six-figure small business strategist for service professionals is to serve marriages, new businesses, stuck and unmotivated individuals, and communities looking to learn how to make healthier life choices, find a purpose, and learn how to use that purpose to live life on their own terms. Sometimes, that means that I am called upon to make sacrifices and to lead from the front lines. The minute I decided that custodial work was beneath me or that I was somehow more privileged than other people, I began living outside that purpose, and I lost the congruence between my core values, vision, and goals. That awareness didn't make the toilet any less stinky or the reality of cleaning it any less gross, but it did serve as a very powerful reminder that I was approaching the task from the entirely wrong perspective.

Ask yourself: Am I living a congruent lifestyle?

A FULL LIFE CAN BE YOURS

One of the most consistent character traits in every successful leader is having the humility to be critiqued and admit error. To truly live a congruent lifestyle, you must first be confident in the soundness of your vision and purpose. No matter how certain you think you are, there is always space to question your beliefs and reasons to learn from others, even within your own family or company.

In my career as a small business strategist and a chiropractor, I have encountered people who tell me that they want to buy something dramatic, thinking that it will bring them happiness and fulfillment. But soon after we work together, it becomes apparent to both of us that they are really trying to avoid the life they have now because it isn't as good as somebody else's. I remember listening to an old-timer chiropractor on an actual cassette tape talk about a conversation he had with another chiropractor he was helping. This second chiropractor was complaining that he didn't have the nice car, big house on the beach, and amazing vacations like the chiropractor who lived across the street from him. The old-timer told him what the rich chiropractor did: work sixty- to eighty-hour weeks, which meant he missed all his kids' baseball games, and never took his wife out on a date because he was always working late. The old-timer asked this younger chiropractor about his kids and his relationship with his wife, and he then revealed the flourishing relationship the family had, along with above-average material goods. Finally, the old-timer asked him a simple question: "Are you willing to sacrifice family for fortune?" While there are ways to have an abundant life with an amazing family, we all have a limited amount of time, and it is important to assign that time to what you value most.

Find someone who will speak to you like the old-timer. They will "tell it like it is" and you can trust they won't be a constant "yes" to whatever you suggest. The people in my most valuable relationships have full authority to help me course correct and let me know when they think I am going down the wrong path, just like Jessica did when she asked me if I prayed before applying for that loan money back in 2019. Don't pay more ignorance tax than necessary; instead, find someone in your life who can speak boldly yet kindly to your ambitions and dreams. On the other side of the coin, stay away from the people who are consistently negative and deflate your enthusiasm and passion. As I decided to become a niche chiropractor in the pediatric and prenatal space and outside of all insurance networks, I had many skeptics. How do you determine who to listen to and who to stay away from? In my opinion, the people who can see your vision and who resonate with your purpose are the ones to keep close. The ones who just see goals, rewards, or short-term benefits are the ones you should keep further away. I know conversations around vision and purpose aren't necessarily first-date normal, but that's why Friday night parties never appealed to me in college or even high school. It's why I wanted to become more than just a chiropractor helping physical ailments; I wanted to help people change on a mental level as well. What I do as a strategist, in my opinion, is just mental chiropractic: I provide bursts of energy designed to get the mind moving in the right direction and hopefully leading to paradigm shift and eventually self-propelled success and abundance.

THE MINDSET OF ABUNDANCE

Everyone, I am sure, can remember March 2020 when the COVID-19 pandemic hit. Schools stopped, transportation stopped, toilet paper ran out, and fear gripped the world. I was just getting back on my feet after nearly losing my business, but I was armed with a new perspective. Instead of seeing fear, I saw opportunity. Even though my bank account was still recovering, I owned the mindset of abundance. Small businesses were hit even harder than I was, and a mentor of mine challenged other people in the community to pay it forward by creating fifty dollar or one hundred dollar tabs at coffee shops and other local places. This not only established goodwill at these local businesses, but they also let me remind other people in my community that I was thinking about them and that I cared for them even when they felt like they were on their own. I still wasn't nearly as far back in the black as I wanted to be, but I put my faith in living in abundance. It worked. The more I invested in others, the more they invested in me. The more I gave, the more people found and joined my practice. I was putting this abundance mindset to the test and found out that, when I live in scarcity, the less I have and the bigger the problems grow. When I live in abundance, however, I receive back more than I sow, and my problems continually shrink. People come out of the woodwork to join my vision and be a part of solving a problem and doing good for others.

I firmly believe that I was able to grow 30 percent through a pandemic year in a shut-down state with a service-based business because of the change in my perspective. Had I done what most other people did (panic, hoard, fight) I believe this book never would have been written, and it's very possible that I would be flipping burgers for a living. The problem was never really my bank account: it was that I had stopped doing what I was called to do and had abandoned the vision I had created. I was acting selfish instead of pursuing a purposeful life as a servant.

The value you give to the world will show in your network, your net worth, and the joy that you have living a life of purpose. When you put out creativity, what comes back to you is the valuation of that creativity. If you tell me your goal is to make money, I'm going to tell you you need to go back to Chapter 1 of this book and really think about your selfless purpose first, and your selfish why second. You should be doing what you are doing because someone is going to suffer if you don't. The same is true whether your goal is losing weight or beginning a new relationship or getting out of debt. This world needs you to think bigger than yourself. There are problems you were put on this earth to solve and people you were created to help. The more we can focus on that, the better this place is for everyone. Instead of fighting for a bigger slice of a small pie, let's work together to make the pie bigger.

...UNTIL YOU MAKE IT

I'm not a big fan of the expression *fake it 'til you make it*. To me, the concept of faking it just seems so fake, and that seems at odds with a congruent lifestyle. Instead, I like the idea of living your aspirations, even before you've fully realized them. There are limits to this, of course, and I am definitely not advocating that you spend beyond your means. Instead, I firmly believe anything that costs you, rather than adds to you over time, is a liability and should be avoided.

I also believe there is real value in embracing the future version of you and that vision you have created. My wife Jess has developed a new love for homesteading and gardening. One of her YouTube mentors said, "Turn your waiting room into a classroom." So even though our property is dry and undeveloped, we decided to homestead where we are and start by getting two pigs. Jess had visions of lush pasture, big gardens, animals everywhere, and living as close to living off the land as possible, but we knew that might not be possible where we are now. So pigs were our way of living in the vision of a homesteader, even though it was just pigs. Let me tell you, this vision is coming true not even a year later on this same property. We now have about twenty chickens, a couple turkeys, seven pigs, 3,000 square feet of garden space, two cows, and the beginnings of a lush green pasture. I'm sure the housing tract in front of us thinks we are nuts, but we are home-steaders in the Southern California desert. Even better, we have a Facebook group with over one hundred other local homestead-ers, from windowsill farmers to market farms, and a community that gets together once per month to share produce, learn new skills, and let our kids play. We didn't fake it, nor have we made it, but getting those two pigs instilled the confidence and desire to continue trying the next thing on the list.

If your goal is to hike the Pacific Crest Trail, go ahead and subscribe to outdoor magazines and buy some of the gear you'll need for the trip. Do small hikes and spend time around people who like hiking. Eventually you will be the mentor teaching the greenhorn the hacks of hiking the PCT. I have a friend who began telling everyone he knew that he was going to compete in a Spartan Race long before he ever registered or was even in shape to race it. For him, the simple act of telling people about his intentions created a commitment he felt he had to make good on. He was a Spartan competitor in his mind before even finishing, but when the race started, he was able to finish and was already looking at the next step up.

Don't be discouraged when people don't yet value you the way you deserve to be. One of my favorite little stories is of a woman who approached a famous artist when he was having dinner at a restaurant. The woman told him how much she loved his work and asked if the artist would make her a quick sketch on a bar napkin. The artist pulled a pen from his jacket pocket and, with a few strokes, obliged her. The woman was elated, but when she reached for the napkin, the artist stopped her.

"Not so fast," he told her. "That'll be $3,000."

The woman was furious. "That took you less than a minute to draw," she responded.

The artist disagreed. He pointed out all the classes he had attended, along with the years of apprentice work and failure. He described the back-breaking hours spent in a cold studio and all the exhibits and shows he had participated in. "This napkin is the representation of a lifetime of work," he told her. "Three thousand dollars is, frankly, a steal."

The biggest asset we can ever invest in is ourselves, but it's also the main thing people carelessly give away. Just because you are new at what you do doesn't mean it is worthless. You have a lifetime of experience, however much that is, and you need to value that or else other people won't either. I will be honest: writing this book was hard. There were so many times I questioned whether I had anything good to say. I am not original, famous, a guru, or the owner of a penthouse in New York, but I am me. As I wrote, I would share with my patients along the way, and it was amazing seeing and hearing the impact it had in their lives. I also knew there were going to be many people just like them who needed to hear this message.

CONCLUSION

My FATHER-IN-LAW RETIRED A FEW YEARS AGO AND STARTED creating and selling hand-crafted farmhouse tables. I've learned a lot about life by watching him in his workshop. With each new project, he'll begin with raw wood that he cuts down to size. Before he can assemble and stain the table, though, he first spends hours sanding down each piece. I've always considered sanding to be total drudgery—on par with having to grate a hundred pounds of carrots with a rusty old vegetable grater. But after doing a few wood projects myself, I've gained a new appreciation for that part of the project. Sanding is a great analogy that we can use in multiple aspects of our lives. I call it *sandpaper moments:* those times when we have the opportunity to be shaped from a raw, jagged person into a smooth, usable, and better version of ourselves. It feels hard to have bits and pieces of us swept away, but it is important to remember that those pieces were actually holding us back and potentially even causing harm to others.

This book is an example of one of my own sandpaper moments. When I began writing it, everything felt like a ton of exhausting work. I'd finish a drafting session exhausted and with the emotional equivalent of bloody knuckles. But as I kept going, the process became more and more manageable. I was transitioning from a super-coarse grit that met with a lot of resistance to a much finer process that took less effort and yielded more refined results. It was kind of like all that friction I felt during my rock bottom moment in 2019, and throughout the years before that, finally allowed me to clarify my purpose and develop the discipline it takes to make that purpose a reality. Instead of letting the sandpaper moments wear you out, persevere through and a better, more refined self will be revealed.

As I stressed in Chapter 4, it is always important to remember that you don't have to tackle any problem alone. I truly believe that my ultimate goal is serving others, particularly when it comes to helping them rewire their brain for success and abundance. I also believe that, once you begin living your selfless purpose, the contributions you have to offer will go a long way toward making the world a better place. That's why I've created a *Perspective* mentorship community, a group where you can find other people struggling to solve their own problems and who are eager to collaborate as a group or simply find encouragement. It's why I continue to offer workshops and lectures with additional lessons on how to create, foster, and grow the collective abundant mindset in the church, in the community, and in the world. Together, we can rise to the occasion so that when we meet friction, we can call upon each other and work collectively to ensure that each generation is better than the one before.

Does it work? Well, every successful person I know and read about gives more than they take. Every successful leader I know serves, rather than makes slaves. Every leader has a vision, a self-less purpose, a selfish why, and goals to make their dreams a reality. Every person that I have met who lives in a state of abundance is ultimately successful because of it.

Creativity is, in my opinion, the defining characteristic of humanity. Think about the oldest living species, and they are still living the same way they did thousands of years ago. I have been alive for thirty-one years on this earth, and I saw the invention of the internet, cell phone, Amazon, Netflix, and so much more. I can't imagine what human creativity will lead to in the next thirty years. Creativity is only possible when you apply the abundant mindset while living in a neurological state of ease and with a strong sense of purpose. You matter, and we need you to show off your creative genius. I am excited that this book can aid you in your journey to pursuing a life of success and abundance.

I am rooting for you.

EPILOGUE

First, I just wanted to say thank you for reading. I am truly honored to have spent this time with you, and I hope this book was a catalyst for you to step into your world-changing purpose. I wanted to make sure I took a few lines here to elaborate on my faith journey, as I mentioned it multiple times throughout the book. I am a believer in the resurrected Jesus, and I claim Him as my Savior. If I am being honest, I believe He is the true source of the abundance mindset, because in Him all things are possible. He is infinitely loving and infinitely creative: two things I want more of day by day. You don't have to act a certain way to talk to Him. He loves you just as you are, and He wants to see His great purpose for humanity manifest in you. I believe this is why we have such a drive to create and help, because the God of the Bible is the Creator and ultimate Helper. We were created in His image; therefore we naturally reflect His characteristics. I want to encourage you in your spiritual walk, and if you feel lost, feel free to reach out and I would be happy to have that conversation.

Second, I know I raise a lot of questions and don't give a lot of answers in this book. I did that on purpose because it requires a bit more of a personal approach and more words than I care to write, so I created a video course expanding on the concepts in this book and hopefully narrowing down your questions you need answered to propel you further. Visit www.drchrisboman. com to learn more.

ACKNOWLEDGMENTS

First, I have to thank my Lord and Savior Jesus Christ. As cliche as it might sound, He truly filled me with years of wisdom as I wrote this book and every concept was, I believe, supernaturally downloaded. There were times I would finish a session and look back on what happened and just be amazed with what came out. This is why I need to get this message out to you, because He had you in mind when He was speaking to me.

Jessica, my beautiful bride, thank you. In the time it took to write this, we had another kid, bought a couple cows, and battled through intense spiritual warfare. You have been with me through the thick and thin, and I want to thank you for encouraging me time and time again. I am excited to see the fruits of your labor through this book touch the lives of many others.

To my chiropractic mentors, thank you. Without a successful chiropractic practice this book doesn't exist. Without the chiropractic lifestyle and philosophy, I would be lost in a back pain practice just waiting to retire.

To my friends, thank you for encouraging my passion and for asking me the right questions. Thank you for challenging me and caring for my heart and my future.

Finally, reader, thank you for picking up this book and making the commitment to live a life of great purpose to experience success and abundance.